"ONE OF THE RARE BOOKS that discusses medical decisions sensibly and, at the same time, attends to their deep emotional components. It is especially useful to people who face critical medical decisions."

> **Albert R. Jonsen, Ph,D.**
> Former Member of The President's Commission
> for the Study of Ethical Problems in Medicine

"FINALLY WE HAVE A HOPE for healing our institutions and the people who work inside them. [This book]... speaks to the wisdom of 'healer, heal thyself.'"

> **Paul Brenner, M.D.**
> Clinical Faculty, Scripps Memorial Hospital
> La Jolla, California
>
> Lecturer, author of *A Shared Creation:*
> *The Meaning of Pregnancy* and
> *Health is a Question of Balance*

The Health Connection

Building Partnerships

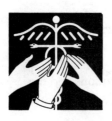

*Empowering
Patients,
Families &
Professionals*

in Hospital Care

MARY DALE SCHELLER, M.S.W.

with the editorial collaboration of Doris Berdahl

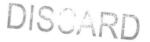

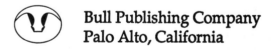

Bull Publishing Company
Palo Alto, California

Copyright © 1988, 1990 by Mary Dale Scheller

Library of Congress Cataloging-in-Publication Data
Scheller, Mary Dale, 1942–
    [Power of 3]
    Building partnerships in hospital care : empowering patients, families & professionals / by Mary Dale Scheller ; with the editorial collaboration of Doris Berdahl.
        p.   cm.
    Reprint. Originally published: The power of 3. Dallas : Saybrook Pub. Co., © 1988.
    Includes bibliographical references.
    Includes index.
    ISBN 0-923521-07-0   : $10.95
    1. Hospital care.   2. Nursing home care.   3. Hospital patients—Family relationships.   4. Nursing home patients—Family relationships.   5. Medical personnel and patient.   I. Berdahl, Doris.
II. Title.
    [DNLM: 1. Family.   2. Hospitalization.   3. Humanism.   4. Professional –Family Relations.   5. Professional–Patient Relations. WX 158.5 S322p 1988a]
RA965.6.S343   1990
362.1'1—dc20
DNLM/DLC   90–2523
for Library of Congress   CIP

Medical, legal and bioethical information changes rapidly and is subject to differing interpretations. Each reader must take responsibility for acquiring current information and processing it carefully both in his or her mind and heart before applying it to specific cases.

Bull Publishing Company   Distributed to the trade by:
P.O. Box 208   Publisher's Group West
Palo Alto, California 94302   4065 Hollis Street
(415) 322-2855   Emeryville, California 94608

Printed in the United States of America

Cover Design: Robb Pawlak
Cover Logo: Ken Miller
Production Manager: Helen O'Donnell
Compositor: Cathy Lombardi

This book is dedicated to:
James Paul Scheller, M.D.
My Care Partner

Table of Contents

Chapter 4
STRENGTHENING THE CARE PARTNERSHIP   67

Some of the deterrents to the care partner approach and ways to handle them: System hierarchy and how to understand it. Hospital rules and what they really mean. Patient rights and how to use them. Power issues and how to constructively assert, blend, and exchange power with others.

Chapter 5
TRANSCENDING THE SYSTEM   103

Ways to bring creativity into the hospital room. The sensory approach: Putting sight, sound, smell, taste, and touch at the service of healing. How to break the rules *with* staff support.

Chapter 6
GIVING without GIVING OUT or GIVING UP   131

How the care partner approach deals with fatigue and "burnout" for both families and professionals. Ways to balance giving and receiving. How to find support—in the community and within institutional walls.

Chapter 7
HANDLING CRITICAL CARE   175

Adapting care partner principles to critical care situations—when the prognosis is for recovery and when it is not. Step-by-step guidance for those readers faced with life-support decisions.

Chapter 8
THE CALL FOR REVOLUTION   215

Vision for the future: A health care system where patients and families are recognized and active members of the hospital health care team. A place where "health care" really means what it says.

Concept Index

For a full understanding of the care partner approach to hospital care, you should read this book from the beginning. But if you are in medical crisis—or if for any reason you require immediate access to specific information—you first may want to turn to material directly related to your needs. With you in mind, I offer what I call my "Concept Index." It should lead you to what you need to know right away.—*MDS*

Acknowledgments

First let me acknowledge Jim Scheller, my husband; Doris Berdahl, my editorial collaborator; David Bull, my publisher; and Gretchen Meinke and Mary Castor, two loyal friends. All of them were sources of support through the long germination and birthing of this book.

Since the mid-1980s, when my manuscript first began to take shape, Doris Berdahl has been intimately involved in its development—not only as a technical advisor and copy editor, but as an active participant in the writing process.

From the beginning, Doris and I developed an unusual team effort. The editing process became a round-robin of response and counter-response until, together, we had honed my first drafts into publishable chapters. Through it all, Doris covered the gamut of editorial chores—from tidying up my spelling and rearranging my commas to acting as midwife to my ideas. As a result her mark is on every page.

My deepest appreciation goes to the entire staff of Bull Publishing Company who saw my vision and wanted to help it become a reality. I am also grateful to Pat Howell of Saybrook Publishing Company who originally suggested the overarching framework and the internal structure which enabled me to translate that vision into text.

Many thanks are in order to my family, friends and professional colleagues, who carefully reviewed and commented on each version of my many manuscripts. Especially I would like to thank my former students at the University of California at Berkeley for launching me on this project. Others who deserve special mention for their ongoing support include Robert Pruger of the University of California at Berkeley, Dennis Jaffe of the Saybrook Institute, and Peter Koestenbaum of San Jose State University.

In addition I would like to thank my friends at the Integral Yoga Institute of San Francisco for the beautiful room they provided for my writing. Every writer should be blessed with such a serene working space, lovingly supplied with fresh fruit and hot tea.

Finally I would like to thank those who first helped me develop these ideas: the staff of the Maury County Hospital; the staff and residents of the Columbia Health Care Facility in Columbia, Tennessee; the staff, patients and care partners of the Planetree Model Hospital Unit in San Francisco; the ministers and members of the First Presbyterian Church of Columbia, Tennessee, and of the Redwoods Presbyterian Church of Larkspur, California. I would especially like to recognize Dr. Carl C. Gardner, Jr., a physician I grew to understand and deeply respect. Moreover, I would like to acknowledge the individual patients, family members and health professionals in numerous institutions who were willing to work with me during these past few years to demonstrate that there *is* a better way of providing care in the hospitals and nursing homes of this country.

Love is to life
As after is to rain;
I've seen it pass through
Birth and death,
Make prism out of pain.
So penetrant a light,
So pure its substance
Seems to be,
All window shutters
Only prove
Their insufficiency.

—Victoria Forrester
"So Penetrant a Light"
A Latch Against the Wind

The Power of 3

MANIFESTO

The ideas in this book are simple ones, based on the way people naturally want to behave when a loved one is ill. Much of what is proposed already takes place to some degree in most American hospitals. *But only after the doctor or nurse has left the room.*

Once alone, family members begin to straighten sheets, adjust pillows, and slip homemade chicken soup out of shopping bags. These are time-honored caring practices. But in the face of modern technology and hospital practices, they've been forced underground.

Many professionals work underground, too. Doctors, nurses, others on the hospital team are sensitive to the emotional and spiritual needs of patients and their families. They listen with understanding to people's fears, their concerns. And, acting in quiet, unofficial ways, they see that those in their charge get what they need—the nightly back-rub, the personally arranged admission to the only sunlit room, the unauthorized permission to extend visiting time just ten minutes more.

Unfortunately, in today's health care environment, this form of care normally occurs *in spite of* the institution, not *because of* it. As a result, family members never are acknowledged for the part they play in the healing process. Caring professionals go unrecognized and unrewarded for going the extra mile. And hospitals miss the chance to publicize the presence of such important services within their walls.

The three-way partnership proposed in this book can change all that. I call it the POWER OF 3. Using this model, a patient, a family member or friend and a health professional, working in concert, can become a dynamic care-giving triad. By combining their strengths and talents, they can extend their effectiveness, heighten their creativity, spread their energy. And ultimately the POWER OF 3, growing exponentially, can achieve small miracles.

The POWER OF 3 is so disarmingly simple, however, that hospitals may tend to underestimate its potential. They would be wise not to do so. With no additional staff, no special training, no extra outlay of money, it can transform rigid institutions, focused solely on curing, into flourishing sanctuaries, committed to curing *and* caring.

Indeed the transformation is already underway. Patients and families are demanding that hospitals be more sensitive to their needs. Doctors, nurses and administrators are actively searching for ways to respond. The POWER OF 3 can show them how.

In fact, it can do far more. It can inspire all of us to work for fundamental reform. By seeking our solutions together rather than apart, we can act in ways that make a profound difference in both the hospital and nursing home experience. By thus drawing on our combined strengths, we can launch a health care revolution.

Chapter 1

THE HOSPITAL ILLNESS
THAT HAS NO NAME

Katherine pushed through the heavy glass doors of the hospital. Her years as a therapist and wife of a doctor should have prepared her for this. The fluorescent pallor of the corridors leading off in every direction and the nylon rustle of nurses passing briskly by to the elevators made it seem like every other hospital she'd ever known. But this one was different. Her father was in one of these rooms, seriously ill. And Katherine, who had calmly ministered to the pain and fright of others, was now in the grip of her own fear.

A familiar scene. Thousands of us go through it each year. All it takes are the old sensory stimulants—the hospital smells in the hall, the crisp starchiness of the doctor's coat, the synthetic swish of the nurse's skirt—to call up the old foreboding, the sense of helplessness, the locked-in feeling of being the only person in the world unprepared to deal with crisis.

3

Consider what happens after Katherine joins her relatives in the family waiting room. The doctor in attendance has joined them.

A tall, balding man, he wore heavy glasses, rimless on the lower half, outlined by dark frames across his brow, giving him the look of a stern father figure. His starched white coat bore his name, neatly stitched across the pocket—Charles R. Lloyd, M.D.

He looked tired, dispirited. His body seemed to be fixed in a permanent stoop. His eyes didn't focus on anyone in particular, but looked through and past all of them. Dr. Lloyd was a man of few words. But now he spoke quickly, deftly, laying out the technical facts and then delivering his diagnosis: an episode of ventricular tachycardia, an arrhythmia of the heart.

Grasping little or nothing of what they'd heard, the family nodded agreement with his conclusions. Surely he knew his job. Taking their mute acquiescence as a sign that he could leave, the doctor moved toward the door.

When medical crisis occurs, we who are most affected by it need to feel we can count on professionals to come to our aid, emotionally as well as medically. But often, just the opposite happens. Those we rely on to minister to us don't have the time or the interpersonal skills to support us in the ways we need. As a result, the hospital experience, which should be a healing one, turns into a painful and dehumanizing ordeal.

Our reaction is often bitter. But what we've failed to realize is that those we're looking to for help are suffering, too. In different ways and for different reasons, doctors have the same locked-in feeling. So do nurses. Whether they're conscious of it or not, *everyone* involved in a health care crisis has the same ominous feeling—from administrators to orderlies, from unit clerks to hospital volunteers. Nobody is immune from it.

And in the end, this foreboding that nobody can define— that few can even acknowledge—succeeds in isolating us from one another. It causes us to become defensive, prevents us from reaching out to one another, keeps us from forming a solid front against the forces that threaten us all.

Follow Katherine and her party through this first day—and try reading their minds.

The family, a pace or two behind the doctor, approached John McGuire's room. Through the open door, they heard a machine, rhythmically beeping and hissing. Entering the room, they saw a motorized bed, surrounded by its satellite system. A square IVAC machine, blinking red when its IV needed changing. A monitor, one end pasted to John's chest, the other to an alert system which would bring nurses flying if the signal came in strange.

Almost lost among the technology was the patient. He wore a wrinkled white hospital gown with "Madison County Hospital" stamped across its front. His eyes were closed, his body pale and still. Tubes were attached to all his orifices. As his family gathered around his bed, it seemed to them that he and this life monitoring machinery had been in mortal conflict—and the machinery had won.

FAMILY MEMBER: . . . *it's all wrong . . . somebody should do something . . . everybody's calm . . . I'm scared . . . blown away . . . glad no one knows how helpless I feel . . .*

DOCTOR: . . . *hope this is quick . . . need to get home before 9 tonight . . . so tired . . . bone tired . . . don't know what's happening here . . . tired of sounding like I do . . . tired of playing God when I'm not . . .*

NURSE: . . . *they're so scared . . . .need someone to talk to . . . not me . . . got chewed out last time . . . my neck as usual . . . staying clear of these people and their problems . . .*

> PATIENT: . . . *wait a minute . . . what about me? . . . flat on my back . . . talking past me like I'm nothing . . . what's wrong with me? . . . gotta get out of here . . . somebody, help me!*

For over twenty years, I've sensed these silent monologues. And I've seen them take their toll. Watched people being assaulted by feelings they've only dimly recognized—or failed to recognize at all—and suffering the consequences of that unawareness. I call it "the hospital illness that has no name."

It's not only all-pervasive, it's like a cancer. It grows. What usually begins as vague, undefined dread almost always becomes something worse—for some people, helplessness and passivity; for others, anger and bitterness. But whatever form the dissatisfaction takes, it seems to stem from one source: the way we provide care in the American hospital system. Institutions designed to offer the finest care in the world, staffed by highly trained professionals acting from the best of intentions and with the finest technology, fail to respond to people's deepest needs.

Why this should be so is puzzling. These needs *seem* so easy to satisfy. *Everyone* needs to be heard and understood. *Everyone* needs to be treated with kindness and respect. But, as simple and universal as these needs are, they remain unmet in a system which continually misses the point. Why?

The answer is simply that our large medical institutions, with their sprawling networks of departments and medical staffs, their nursing hierarchies and specialized services, their teaching programs and outpatient clinics, have lost sight of how human beings want to give and receive care. Operating in a universe of their own making, they have set in motion a destructive force, one that not only fails to give healing care, but brings out the worst in everyone connected with it.

6

Patients cut off from loved ones, assigned tiny cubicles in faceless rooms, feel isolated and depersonalized. Family members, refused a significant role in the care program, feel ignored and depreciated. Professional and administrative staff, overworked and unrecognized, suffer emotionally and become disenchanted with their work. In consequence, all parties retreat behind their own lines, unwilling to speak about their personal pain and confusion and unable to invite such revelations from others. The result: mutual misunderstanding and lack of compassion for each other's plight.

It didn't take long for Katherine and her family to become part of this world. They watched from the sidelines while scores of strangers worked on their loved one—almost always without their participation, usually without their full understanding, sometimes without their knowledge. Doctors, nurses, LVNs and orderlies followed a time-honored medical practice—doing what they felt they had to do, and hoping the family would leave them alone to get on with it. The results were negative for everyone.

The family caught the doctor in the hall during his evening rounds. Though their questions were reasonable enough, their looks were the ones doctors dread. Their mouths asked, "What's his temperature? Is he responding?" But their body language pleaded, "He will live, won't he? You will do something so he won't die? Please fix him. Or at least tell us you will!"

In other words, what they were saying gave little hint of what they were thinking and feeling. It may have gone like this.

FAMILY MEMBER I: *. . . so jumpy, so scared . . . can't make out what the doctor's saying . . . wish he'd make me feel better . . . why's this happening to me? . . .*

FAMILY MEMBER II: . . . *that doctor's not leveling with us . . . knows something we don't know . . . isn't telling us the whole truth . . . well, we've got rights . . . we don't have to take this from anyone. . .*

DOCTOR: . . . *got to be careful here . . . not much chance for the patient . . . but not about to tell them now . . . he could pull through . . . better wait and see . . .*

NURSE: . . . *questions, questions, questions . . . never going to finish my work . . . need to get through before shift change . . .*

PATIENT: *What about me? . . . am I just something incidental here?*

Confusion, denial, self-doubt, defensiveness, resentment, distrust. All are attitudes that can undermine and ultimately destroy the chance of these people working together on the care, and possible recovery, of this patient. Surely there's a better way. In fact, there is. I've seen other approaches tried. I know there are alternatives that work. There *are* ways to conquer "the hospital illness that has no name."

Since 1983, when I first experimented with some of these methods, I've been convinced that any patient, family member or health professional can choose to end this perceived victimization by the hospital and nursing home system. In fact, they can go further. They can make the hospital experience a time of enrichment, renewal and personal growth. I've begun to develop such a program, one that can be launched simply, naturally and less expensively than any form of care in use at the present time.

Yet the tendency of most of us is to wait for institutions to change on their own. But institutions don't change, individuals change. So my method relies on the individual, on one person or a small group of persons at any rung in the hospital or nursing home hierarchy to take the initiative to act—and then to mobilize others to do the same. It *can* happen. I've seen extraordinary change occur when people like us are given the idea and the support to do what is already in our better nature to do. We can make a difference. That's what this book is about. That's what the Planetree experiment is about.

The Planetree Model Hospital Unit, located on the top floor of Pacific Presbyterian Medical Center in San Francisco, is a pilot project for exploring more humanistic approaches to hospital care. In the summer of 1985, I asked Planetree to allow me to test the efficacy of a simple idea. I wanted to see whether the instinct to look after loved ones in times of crisis could translate into serious lay participation in a hospital care program. It was a radical idea. But Planetree was trying radical ideas.

An architect had completely redesigned a medical unit on the 6th floor. Patients' rooms had been remodeled. Soft natural colors had replaced the standard hospital orange. Oak cabinets had banished the stainless steel carts. Track lighting had taken over from the fluorescent tube. Original paintings had been bought or borrowed from local museums and hung with care. Audio cassettes had been purchased so that patients could relax with music of their own choice.

The nurses' station, which had previously acted as a barrier between staff and patients, had been removed. A kitchenette had been provided for the use of family members, where they could prepare favorite meals for their loved ones. A patient lounge had been created, not just for socialization and education, but for occasional live entertainment—a place where TV and VCR could sometimes be replaced by musicians brought in from the outside.

Every patient was to have a primary nurse. Rather than ever-changing teams of nurses, a single individual would be responsible to and for the patient, serving not only as care-giver but also as advocate, health educator and friend. The patient's at-home schedule was to be honored; and visitors were to be admitted at any time at the patient's request. The patient was to be given the option of learning about his prescribed medications from the primary nurse, after which drug administration could become his responsibility. And in the most radical departure of all, the patient was to have access to the medical chart and could not only read it, but write in it.

But the program, while remarkably innovative, needed one more component to make it complete—a partnership between the patient, the family and the hospital. Its founder had envisioned something of the kind, but little had been done yet to implement it. And for good reason. Of all the Planetree experiments, it would require perhaps the most radical shift from the way hospitals traditionally do business.

Moreover, "conventional wisdom" said it couldn't be done. For one thing, it would have to rely on participants with no medical background, working side-by-side with profes-sionals. For another, it would have to take place in an en-trenched, highly complex and technical environment. Finally, and most important, it would require everyone involved to adopt new attitudes and behaviors.

But I believed it could work. And it has. Here's how it was originally conceived—and how, with some modifications, it has evolved at Planetree and other hospitals where I've consulted.

The structure is a three-way partnership, in which the patient and family members and/or friends join health profes-sionals in becoming active and recognized members of the hospital health care team. In this partnership, the professionals are teachers to the patient and family in the area of physical care. But the patient and family are teachers to the professional staff in that other, equally important realm—emotional, social and spiritual care, delivered in a form suited to *that* patient's healing process. The program centers on the patient as the director of the team. In cases where the patient is too ill to participate, the patient designates one of the caregivers as primary spokesperson.

The team members are encouraged to come out in the open about their needs and feelings; and, conversely, to be honest about their capabilities and limitations in filling the needs of others. Most important, they are asked to tap the wellspring of emotional energy they share with all human beings—and use that precious resource to care for one another.

At first, all this was only a concept. But since then, it has come to be known as "care partnering"—an idea whose timeliness has now been demonstrated.

During Planetree's very first year, individuals without special medical background and with no special penchant for self-sacrifice put the concept into practice. A retired grocery-man learned to do extensive nursing for his wife, who was suffering from amyotrophic lateral sclerosis (Lou Gehrig's disease). He monitored her ventilator and feeding bag, cleaned her gastric tube, suctioned her trachea and administered her medications.

"I never knew I could learn this much," he said after the first few days. "It makes me feel so self-sufficient." When he took a break from the Planetree unit, he was the one who left written directions on the nursing care to be done. And when his wife was discharged home, he was well trained and ready to assume full responsibility for her care.

11

Other lay people on the unit learned how to apply compresses, give baths, change dressings, flush catheters, give medication, and take temperatures and blood pressures.

Some did only psycho-social care, the kind of nursing that comes naturally to family and close friends—if they can feel comfortable and supported while doing it. "What's really important," said one care partner, "is seeing that Joe has catsup on his eggs and brown sugar for his cereal. That's what he would have at home."

Nurses reported how often people's personalities changed when they became care partners. "One family member used to sit around the ward and mope. Her state of mind and her physical condition were really going downhill," a nurse told me. "But when she became useful, both her self-esteem and her health improved almost overnight."

Care partnering actually pulled people out of despair. An AIDS patient at Planetree and his care partner, instead of brooding about what lay ahead, decided to leave a gift for future patients. First they redecorated the bathroom of the patient's suite with a colorful shower curtain and poster for the next person to enjoy. Then, upon discharge, they offered to send bright shower curtains and posters for every bathroom on the unit as an act of appreciation for their extraordinary care.

In other words, Planetree demonstrations provided proof of an old truism we too often forget: When we can work *with* a system instead of *against* it, all kinds of creative energies are unleashed that work in everybody's best interests.

The following chapters show how you can unleash these energies during any stage in the hospital experience and on any unit of the institution—from pediatrics to geriatrics, from obstretics to critical care. The book will take you step-by-step through the creation of your own care partner program, one custom-tailored to your needs and personal style. Some of the information is directed at professionals who want to institute care partnering on specific units of their hospitals or in their nursing home settings; some to administrators who want to adopt the program throughout entire medical centers. Some is aimed at patients and family members interested in creating their own programs, with or without institutional backing and support.

My hope is that each reader will be inspired to introduce into any hospital or nursing home at least one idea suggested here. Hopefully several. The secret lies in making many small moves forward. A cumulative effort can become the basis of fundamental hospital reform. In essence, the POWER OF 3 can become the power of thousands. I'm convinced through our combined effort, we *can* cure "the hospital illness that has no name."

Chapter 2

MAKING CHOICES

CHOICES WITHIN OURSELVES

Katherine walked down what seemed an interminable hallway and passed through some heavy double doors. Propelled by an urgent need to be with her father, she headed for the Coronary Care Unit, alone and unauthorized.

She sensed a quickening of her pulse. She realized her hands were trembling. But walking had mobilized her energy and strengthened her resolve. She knew that what she was doing was right for her.

Walking up to the nurses' station, she said, "I think the best thing right now is for me to be with my father."

Taken by surprise, uncertain how to respond, they stared at her wordlessly. And that moment of hesitation gave her the chance she needed. She used it to walk directly into her father's room.

The first issue to be resolved when the possibility of a relationship with a sick person arises is whether the family member or friend in question really *wants* to do this and, if so, to what extent. Because of the challenging nature of that experience—of being with an ill or impaired person—an even more appropriate question might be: Does that person really *need* to have such a relationship—not with just anyone, but with *this* patient at this particular time?

In the scene above, Katherine, driven by a compelling need, has overcome her fear of hospital authority and moved decisively to do what she *must* do—minister to her father. Another daughter (wife, brother, friend), equally loving and concerned, might not feel that need—and, if she doesn't, she shouldn't.

The point is that care partnering, as I'm defining it here, is completely optional. Everybody involved—patient, family member, professional—gets to say "yes" or "no."

Coming Clean

When I've worked as care partner facilitator at Planetree, and as consultant to other hospitals, I've begun by asking questions. A lot of questions. As many as it takes to get at the truth: that is, whether the primary parties to this agreement—the health professional, the patient and the family member/friend—are prepared to make a serious commitment, one from the heart. The essential element in these negotiations is honesty, a willingness by everybody to come clean—without equivocation or self-delusion, and especially without guilt.

If there's no facilitator working with them, they can conduct these negotiations on their own. But if there is one, all the better. Let's assume there is. The facilitator begins by questioning each party separately. And in some cases, once the truth is known, imagined barriers disappear.

> DOCTOR: It's an interesting theory. But I'm not convinced it's practical. I'm just too busy to give it the time it would need.
>
> NURSE: I'd really like to try it. I think it could work. But I'd be getting over onto the doctor's turf. And I don't think he'd go for that.
>
> FACILITATOR: No problem. Have the patient ask that his nurse, rather than his doctor, be the professional involved. And those instructions can be written right into his chart.

When this seeming impasse is handled in this manner the doctor, who frankly admits he can't make the commitment, is off the hook. And the nurse, who feels she can, doesn't have to worry that she's overstepping her bounds. In fact, with this approach the patient is free to ask any professional within the hospital walls to serve in the care partner triad.

Where the questioning is focused on a patient and family member, again the object is to get the parties to acknowledge and articulate needs and desires. But truth telling is especially difficult in such cases. These relationships may carry too much emotional baggage for candor to come easily. Here are some of the ways truth is evaded.

> PATIENT I: If my wife wants to take care of me, I guess I should let her. I don't feel much like talking to anyone, but I know it would give her pleasure and I hate to deny her that.
>
> PATIENT II: I'd really like my daughter to be here with me, but I'm afraid it would be an imposition on her. She has so many demands on her already. Better not ask.

In responding to Patient I, the job of the facilitator is to get him to declare outright, "Look, I don't want my wife here. I just want to be left alone." If and when he does, the facilitator should lend immediate support to this honest statement of fact. It should be emphasized that the patient has as much right to refuse a care partner program as to choose one.

To resolve the uncertainty and guilt of Patient II, the facilitator must get to the only person who can effectively do that, the daughter. In a separate interview, the question should be posed simply and directly: does she or doesn't she want to become involved? A variety of replies are possible. The least helpful is some variation on:

> DAUGHTER: I'd like to get involved, but I have a husband and three children to look after. Then there's my part-time job and the PTA auction coming up . . .

In these situations, few phrases more readily signal trouble than "I'd like to get involved, but . . ." In fact, any response that includes "but" should be scrutinized closely, as well as the string of "good reasons" that usually accompany it. How much better if this discussion had begun and ended like this:

> FACILITATOR: Are you interested in becoming part of the hospital care team? For a specified number of hours, you'd be responsible for a certain number of tasks which we—you and I and your father—would decide ahead of time.
>
> DAUGHTER: No, I'm just not comfortable in hospitals and it's not quite right for me to take this on now.

By not equivocating, this daughter has saved everyone time and trouble, including herself. People need to feel as comfortable as possible in the caring role, especially within the hospital/nursing home, where caring provided by families is indeed a choice.

Before entering a care partnership, we should weigh our other commitments and responsibilities. We should look at our emotional strengths at this time in our lives. We should assess whether we'd rather make our contribution inside the hospital or outside it. And finally, if we've chosen to become involved, we should schedule time for our own rest and relaxation.

When Katherine and her family decided to set up their own, informal care partner program, some members felt powerfully drawn to the idea. Some did not.

It took the children of the family a while to realize that their mother, who had been a "take charge" person all her life, was turning their father's care over to them. Agnes McGuire had always had an aversion to hospitals and nursing homes. And now, the idea of long stretches in a sick room, even by the side of her beloved husband, had further stiffened her resistance. A short high-energy woman of 66 with a full head of pure white hair, she came from a long line of strong-willed southern women who believed that people—even sick ones—shouldn't ask for more help than they absolutely need. For the most part, they should tough it out on their own.

So those family members who wanted to try care partnering—Katherine and her sister-in-law, Sarah—were given a tacit go-ahead by those family members who didn't—Agnes and her son Teddy.

"Do you still have those notes you've been keeping?" Sarah asked Katherine on the second day of John's confinement.

Katherine fished in her purse and brought out her airline boarding pass, where she'd been jotting notes since her arrival. Scribbled around the margins and down the back of the small scrap of paper were the doctor's diagnosis and some of her own thoughts and observations.

"Looks like you're running out of space," Sarah said. "What would you think about buying a decent notebook and keeping our own nursing journal?"

Katherine shot a surprised look at Sarah, as if in sudden recognition of something she'd known all along. For the past 48 hours she'd been trying to pin down an idea that kept trying to take shape in her head. Of course! That was it! A kind of hospice program where the family, instead of caring for John at home, would do it right in the hospital.

Propelled by the simple power of this idea, the McGuire family began to close ranks. Plans were laid to get permission for Katherine and Sarah to sleep over in John's room, to learn some simple nursing tasks, to make their own observations and record them in their log.

Agnes, though still unconvinced, volunteered to have hot meals ready for them when they came home for breaks. Teddy said he'd start work on the insurance forms.

So without benefit of a facilitator, this family, while fundamentally divided, struck a workable bargain. A clear division of labor was established. A care partner program, while they didn't call it that, was launched.

How Much is Too Much?

"We're asking you to trust our instincts. We think we can give Dad what he needs most now—emotional and spiritual support. But we can't do it unless we have your support."

With this opening, Katherine had managed to get Dr. Lloyd's attention, but it clearly wasn't getting her much else. He'd already begun shaking his head. Whatever she was going to ask, his look seemed to say, the answer would be "no."

For the first time since they'd met, Katherine noticed they were about the same height. Moving closer to further engage him, she delivered her bombshell.

"What we want is permission to sleep overnight in the Coronary Care Unit, and we need you to write the order."

Dr. Lloyd backed away from her, a look of incredulity on his face. But she persisted. "The same cot I've been using in the hall could be fitted under the window. There'd be plenty of room for staff to pass between it and the bed. I've already measured the space." In the pause that followed, she added, "We wouldn't interfere with the nurses in any way. You can count on that."

Maybe it was the sheer audacity of her request. Maybe it was the lack of a really good reason to deny her—now that the space problem had been eliminated. Whatever it was, he turned on his heels and started down the hall toward the nurses' station. At first she thought it was all over. He wasn't going to go for it. But a few steps later, his back still to her, he said loud enough for her to hear, "Well, I guess I'd better go prepare the nurses for the shock."

In the absence of a care partner program, the McGuires had to get what they wanted through a series of ad hoc negotiations with their doctor. That placed the family in the position of having to initiate, and the doctor having to respond, every time a new issue came up. A far better way would have been to have established, from the beginning, a set of ground rules for everyone. Questions about the amount of time and effort the care partner is prepared to give, how much the patient is ready to receive, and to what extent the professionals want to participate are then best dealt with through an agreement.

During the first implementation year at Planetree, we set up a written agreement which allowed all parties to specify the limits of their involvement. Prior to entering the agreement, the patient, care partner and health professional discussed how each saw the care plan evolving: what their respective roles would be; when the care would take place and for how long; what kinds of tasks would be involved; who would be responsible for the training; how the plan could be changed when it no longer fit the parties' needs; and when the care partner would take time off to rest.

A typical care partner agreement looked something like the one appearing on the opposite page.

In this agreement Susan Stamps, the primary nurse, assumes responsibility for teaching and supervising Marian Youngman, the wife, in proper methods of nursing care —transferring patient to wheelchair, taking temperatures, giving medications—in exactly the same way she would instruct and monitor a student nurse. During this instruction, Susan acts not only as trainer, but as mentor as well, encouraging and supporting Marian during the learning process.

In the realm of psycho-social care, the patient and care partner take the lead. They let the hospital staff know what kinds of additional support—psychological, social or spiritual—will be most healing for this particular patient. In the Youngmans' case, they explain their use of their Pachelbel tape and their visualization practice. While staff need not participate in these techniques unless they choose to, they *are* required to respect the Youngmans' ideas and provide uninterrupted time for their practice.

22

CARE PARTNER AGREEMENT

PATIENT: Jack Youngman
DIAGNOSIS: Cerebral Vascular Accident (Stroke)
CARE PARTNER: Marian Youngman
RELATIONSHIP TO PATIENT: Wife
PRIMARY NURSE: Susan Stamps, R.N.
CARE PARTNER'S AVAILABLE DAYS: Week days
CARE PARTNER'S AVAILABLE HOURS: 10:00 A.M. - 2:00 P.M.
CARE PARTNER'S PLAN FOR REST AND RESPITE: Wednesday appointment with hairdresser
PATIENT'S PLAN FOR CARE PARTNER(S) CARE: To be determined

CARE PARTNER TASKS:	PERSON RESPONSIBLE	TRAINING COMPLETED	
Monitor medications	Marian Youngman	S.S.	1/14/86
Take temperature	"	S.S.	1/15/86
Take blood pressure	"	S.S.	1/15/86
Give short wheelchair trips	"	S.S.	1/16/86
Assist with lunch	"	S.S.	1/16/86
Listen to Pachelbel's Canon in D Major at 11 A.M.	Jack Youngman/ Marian Youngman	J.Y./ M.Y.	1/16/86
Practice imaging, concentrating healing on the right side	Jack Youngman/ Marian Youngman	J.Y./ M.Y.	1/16/86

Honesty as a Gift

When people can begin to level with each other about what is really important to them and what they can and cannot do, creativity and spontaneity can flow from the care partner process. For example, when nurses find themselves overextended, they can ask for a new approach. When patients feel their needs are not being met, they can say so. When care partners have doubts about their commitment, they can admit it.

> CARE PARTNER: I'm so tired. I just don't feel like being here today.
> PATIENT: Sounds fine to me. Just go home and read a good book.
> NURSE: We'll manage fine. I'll give the medications this morning. And I'll get someone to set up your husband's tape at 11:00.

With the care partner approach, everyone learns that *giving sometimes consists of not giving.* By not giving when it doesn't feel right, you signal that the recipient can count on your honesty. In essence, you send this message: When requests are made that I can't wholeheartedly meet, I'll simply say "no."

Those who must ask for help are far better served by such frankness. They're given permission to make bold and imaginative requests, to rely heavily on friendships, and to slip comfortably into the role of receiver—knowing they can never impose on someone who refuses, gently but firmly, to allow that to happen.

The outcome, too, is usually far more satisfying. When people are allowed to choose only what they want and need to do, quality time in the hospital or nursing home room is ensured. Each party becomes free to be fully present with the other.

Getting Down to Specifics

Besides being honest, the next most important thing for a care partner to be is specific. Everyone has some constraints. Most potential care partners face what seem like insurmountable obstacles—job obligations, family responsibilities, personal health problems, inadequate transportation. But if they limit their care partner commitment to specific tasks and times, they should be able to devise an action plan which they can honor.

> CARE PARTNER I: I can be with Tom on Tuesday and Thursday from 5 to 7 P.M. He and I used to play a lot of tennis together. I guess the best thing I could do for him, if he feels like it, is sit and rap about matches we've been in together.

> CARE PARTNER II: I'll come Saturday afternoon. John asked me to bring him his mail. Letters from friends will cheer him up. And he may need to pay some bills.

Some of the best care partner plans involve help rendered outside the hospital.

> CARE PARTNER III: As I see it, the best thing I could do is walk Margaret's dog every day. I'm walking my own anyway. Taking along Trident isn't that much more trouble.

> CARE PARTNER IV: The greatest need I see is feeding Elizabeth's family. They can get along on TV dinners

most of the time, I guess. But on, say, Wednesdays and
Fridays, a home cooked meal should really hit the spot.

At Planetree, patients are asked to say, as specifically as
possible, what they want. Care partners are helped to make
suggestions and solicit the patient's approval. The nurse is
told of the plan and invited to make suggestions. Once all
three parties agree, the care partner plan is placed in the
medical chart. This allows others on the hospital team to
know what's happening and elevates the care partner plan to
the same status as other therapeutic plans, such as nursing or
physical therapy.

Some families prefer not to have a written plan and that,
too, is their choice. But in those cases the verbal agreement
should be summarized by the nurse or other professional on
the team and placed in the chart or the nursing care plan. If it
isn't, other members of the hospital staff can't respond to the
patient's wishes in an informed way.

Handled in this way, the care partner plan has the
potential for saving time and effort for everyone. It allows
each person involved to do the tasks she wants to do. It allows
each to set limits on what he is willing and able to do. It gives
everyone some indication of what to count on. The care
partner knows that the doctor has only five minutes to spend
on each patient during evening rounds. The nurse knows that
the care partner won't be available to give medications in the
early morning or on Wednesdays. The family knows that the
nurse doesn't care to join them in their daily Bible reading.
The patient knows of his right to limit the degree of care
partner involvement.

PATIENT: I realize my mother flew all the way from
Nebraska to take care of me. And there are helpful things
she can do. She can come in the late mornings, for

instance, water my plants, and eat lunch with me. But I
need quiet in the afternoons and evenings. She should
plan on shopping or sightseeing then.

The fact that the patient felt free to say this resolved a lot
of issues in this case. The mother was able to feel useful. The
daughter got the family support she needed, but only to the
degree she wanted. And the nurse didn't have to mediate a
mother-daughter standoff.

Lack of specificity leaves everyone drained and depleted.
The caregiver either feels resentment at having done "too
much," or worries that she could have done more. The patient
wonders what the caregiver is willing to do, and ends with
vague disappointment at what is actually done. Professionals
try to work with undefined lay involvement, and end by
banishing families from the hospital altogether. Nobody has
anything tangible by which to measure his commitment—or
to savor his achievements. The care partner program corrects
these flaws.

Making Up the Rules

During the first year at Planetree, when the nurses asked
me to draw up rules for carrying out this program on their
unit, I urged that the program be kept flexible to the needs of
the parties involved. In other words, the people most affected
should make up the rules.

For example, one patient may choose to be his own care
partner. He may have no family, or he may be more creative
and resourceful than anyone he could choose. Another patient
may want five or more relatives and friends to alternate
responsibilities. The same may be true of his choice of a

professional partner. That slot might be filled by one or several people. Whatever arrangement feels right and seems to work should be what is used.

The important point is this: The concept of the POWER OF 3 is not a concept of numbers, but of functions. It works because the patient's autonomy, rights and preferences are honored. Since the patient is often too weak to carry out his own wishes, the person he feels closest to does it for him, functioning as his representative. Since patients and family members are usually not familiar with the institution and its ways of operating, the professional handles the job of dealing with the system, functioning as translator and advocate throughout the hospital/nursing home network. But the primary object of everyone is to support and carry out the patient's wishes.

Picking Out the Partners

For the first time since she'd been home, Katherine was back in the church of her childhood. Entering by a side door on a cold Tuesday morning in December, she heard the sound of her footsteps bounced off bare walls and echoed through empty rooms. But as she paused in the winter gloom, reassuring memories flooded back. The smell of the old gas heater in the vestry. The taste of glazed doughnuts after Sunday school. The sound of children's voices in the choir loft.

Wrapping her coat closer, Katherine reminded herself that this was thirty years later. The gas heater had gone cold. The doughnuts had run out. And the child in the choir loft was no more.

"I need a friend," she said as she sank into the deep leather chair in the pastor's study. "Someone who'll support me and tell other people in the hospital what I want for my father." Struggling to express what had brought her there, she began to picture the kind of

person she needed. Someone with a medical education who could give her information. But more than that. Someone with a strong psychological and spiritual base who could understand her fears and guide her aspirations.

"This person doesn't have to be a heart specialist, doesn't even have to be a doctor," she told Reverend Bingham. "A nurse would do just as well, maybe better. It must be someone who'll listen to my fears and beliefs without running away. But someone who'll set me straight if my ideas get too off base—too far from medical reality."

Katherine, while she didn't know it, was describing the ideal candidate for care partnering—the perfect professional for the care partner triad. The professional serving the triad need not be the attending physician—in many cases, *should* not be. The person chosen—preferably by the patient—can be a nurse, another physician in the hospital, a physical therapist, social worker, chaplain, administrator, anyone in the institution who can translate the care partner concept and the wishes of that particular patient to other staff. For that reason, it works best if the professional in the triad is on staff of the institution where the patient is housed. A family member or friend who is also a doctor or nurse—but who is attached to another institution—is better cast in the family care partner role. The professional position should be reserved for someone who can command the attention of colleagues and help lay members of the team through the intricacies of the institution where the care partnering is actually taking place. That person should also be someone whose work schedule keeps him or her in the hospital most of the time.

Some patients pick out their care partners before entering the hospital. Some ask others for recommendations. Some make their selections after admission. They choose from the nurses, therapists, aides they meet on their first day. At Planetree, the primary nurse automatically becomes the professional member on the team; but the patient still has the right to look around for others better suited. The main point in any institution is for the patient to exercise his option to choose.

Care partnering works best when the different parties have a special liking for one another. I've heard a patient say this to her nurse, "I really like the way you do your work. And for some reason, I feel especially close to you. Would you be willing to be on my care partner team?" When this occurs, something important happens for the nurse, the social worker, or the technician who's chosen. It feels good to be noticed, to stand out and be recognized. It feels good to be special.

Being Special

One of the secrets to the success of the care partner program is the principle that each party is special, and therefore will be treated as special by the other members of the team. This concept is extremely important for those patients, family members and staff who must live and work in large, complex and highly impersonal hospital systems.

A common reason for the "hospital illness that has no name" is that no one within modern hospital/nursing home systems really feels cared for. This may seem puzzling to some. Doctors, nurses, social workers, therapists argue that they care for patients day and night. Supervisors point out that they care for their staff. So why is there this sense that nobody cares?

30

Henri Nouwen, in his book *The Wounded Healer*, explains that for a person to really feel cared for, the person must feel that the healer is "forgetting the many for the one." Obviously, this can't be done within a doctor's general practice or in the normal course of a nurse's shift. But within a care partner program, the professional selected and the professional who chooses to serve is *free* and is *encouraged* to do everything possible to treat this patient and this patient's family as different and special—set apart from other patients in his or her care. And the patient and family member are encouraged to treat the staff person that way too.

The effect of such treatment is potent therapy. It's what patients remember long after the hospital experience is over. It's what family members tell their neighbors and friends about. It's what renews rather than depletes professionals.

And it's all so very simple. When people are treated in a special way, they begin to feel special. And when they feel special, health and renewal usually follow.

CHOICES WITHIN THE FAMILY

At home Agnes and Katherine sat for a long time in the family room—the mother on the white wicker couch with the olive green and white striped cushions, the daughter in the white wicker rocking chair. All the furniture was from their past, the wicker pieces originally a gift from a great aunt on the Campbell side. As she rocked, it seemed to Katherine as if these ancestors, the former owners of this house and its furnishings, were there with them—parties to what she knew was about to be discussed. The fact that John McGuire had been in a coma now for three days.

31

Agnes spoke first. "I don't see how this can go on much longer. I'm not sure I can take much more of it." Temporarily reeling, her strength sapped by the unfamiliarity of a husband barely hanging on, this earthy, robust woman, ordinarily so full of life, had retreated inside herself. For the first time in their life together, she'd turned her power over to her children.

But now the old assertion was rekindling. She looked straight at Katherine, fastening her daughter with bold blue eyes, and said, "I wish John would just die. He wouldn't want to go on like this. And we shouldn't make him."

Katherine stopped rocking. She held Agnes's gaze for a second, then broke away from it and looked down at the floor. When she commenced rocking again, the old rockers pounded the bare hardwood with a fierce and driving force.

Medical crisis has a way of exposing the hidden tensions that pull and tug within most families. So when important medical decisions must be made, and especially when families are denied a significant role in the hospital care program, open conflicts tend to erupt.

> FAMILY MEMBER I: We should put Grandma in a nursing home. You're being unrealistic as usual. She can't live by herself any longer.
>
> FAMILY MEMBER II: I'll never put her away. You don't have any regard for her feelings. You never have.

When families feel helpless in the hospital environment, health care choices often provide them with excuses to score points off one another. A flesh-and-blood sister, mother or in-law is a target much more easily seen and besieged than an abstract system. The lesson to be learned from this is clear.

When family members aren't given, or do not acquire, a role (and therefore a power base) within the institution, they're apt to seek power within their own ranks—taking it away from whatever relative is most vulnerable, sometimes the patient.

Winners and Losers

The winner in these showdowns is usually the person who is loudest and most intimidating. Most people rise to crisis by marshalling their resources in ways that have worked for them in the past. So it's not unusual for a group of close relatives—adults in their forties and fifties, or beyond, who have not lived near one another for many years—to reassume the family roles of their childhood. They fall naturally and unconsciously into their old personae—the "responsible child," the "favorite," the "baby," the "black sheep," the "prodigal son."

It's the "out-of-towner" that doctors talk about most. "I'll be working with a family for days, maybe weeks or years," one internist told me, "setting forth a treatment plan that we all agree on. Then someone I've never heard of invades us from Kalamazoo. And, you can count on the fact, he'll want to get involved, get things messed up and cause a lot of trouble." Sometimes whole families—brothers, sisters, spouses, maiden aunts—line up on one side or the other of the disputed issue. And what ensues, depending on the personalities involved, is either an active tug-of-war or a quiet, but vicious stalemate.

Katherine and her mother were in the opening stages of such a struggle, demonstrating a principle familiar to most health professionals who have dealt with the "polarization

33

mode." That is, if there have been strains within a family in the past, they will most likely reassert themselves during medical crisis, often in exaggerated forms. Sometimes this leads to open warfare.

"My experience with families making critical care decisions in hospitals is usually unpleasant," a doctor once remarked to me. "I see a lot of squabbling and mutual hostility among children. They seem to use these decisions as extensions of long-standing family feuds."

But through a care partner program or something like it, things can be different. When family members are treated with respect, they're more likely to treat others with respect. When they're given status and responsibility within the institutional structure, they no longer need to wrest power from anywhere else. They already have it in another, much more important form—in a significant and recognized role on the health care team.

Strategies for Families

Some hospitals and nursing homes are starting family support groups where people can discuss issues important to them. These offer opportunities for care partners to talk about their family dynamics and how to improve them.

During crisis, families are almost always operating under conditions of fear, emotional and physical pain, frustration and fatigue. But as difficult as they are, these times offer opportunities and options. You can choose less effective or more effective ways of dealing with family differences. Here are some suggestions.

- *Be honest about how you feel.* At the same time, keep in mind each other's special sensitivities and feelings.

- *Continue to talk to one another,* regardless of your differences. When you can no longer talk, write letters, even if you're living in the same house. Letters can sometimes express feelings more accurately and be more easily received than verbal communication.

- *Resist drawing non-family members into the battle* against their will or without their knowledge.

- When outsiders *are* invited in with their consent—for instance, professionals in care partner arrangements—*let them know what role you want them to play.* You can ask them to be a listener, mediator, facilitator, educator or advisor. But if they find themselves uncomfortable in their assigned role, give them permission to refuse, change or discontinue it.

- *Put as much energy into caring for the family as for the patient.* Remember, in a way *everyone* is the patient.

CHOICES AMONG PROFESSIONALS

Katherine looked out the window at the darkness below. It had been a long day. People had streamed in and out of her father's room since early morning. An army of new faces over the past 24 hours, turning him, taking his temperature, suctioning him, checking and rechecking the gleaming equipment that was keeping him alive.

Down in the parking area, the night shift was arriving. Lines of cars, their headlights just switching on, filed slowly through the parking lot, those coming in replacing those going out.

A middle-aged nurse, tall and rangy with cropped gray hair, appeared at the door. Nobody Katherine had ever seen before. "I'm Evelyn," she said. "I'll be taking care of Mr. McGuire tonight." Putting on her glasses, she opened a chart she was carrying and turned the pages, looking for something.

"O.K., here it is. He gets turned every two hours." She glanced at Katherine curiously. "Are you his daughter?"

The little energy Katherine had left drained away. She'd told her story to at least four different nurses and technicians that day. She wasn't up for repeating it—explaining again what she'd noticed about her father's turnings. How if you propped him at a certain angle on his side, his labored, erratic breathing would suddenly stop and become smooth and regular.

Working with her back to Katherine, the nurse remarked, "You look tired."

"I guess I'm just tired of dealing with so many people."

Evelyn whirled around full face, her eyes flashing through her reading glasses.

"You got it," she declared. "That's what's the matter around here. I hate this nursing schedule we're on. Different patients everyday. I'd like to stick with a few and get to know them."

She tucked the chart under her arm and put her glasses in her pocket.

"But what can you do? Nurses don't have much say around here. Administration decides, and that's it."

This nurse felt she had no options. External forces beyond her control—in her view, an all-powerful administration —had made arbitrary decisions which dictated how she functioned as a professional.

She had no way of knowing that at that moment a weary administrator was sitting at his desk downstairs, grappling with the problem of meeting his monthly payroll—and not entirely sure he was going to make it.

36

Cuts in federal health programs and new insurance regulations had reduced his revenues by a fourth. Medicare's new way of reimbursing hospitals—at a fixed rate according to diagnosis—was sending patients home much sooner. So those who went left empty beds. And those who stayed were much sicker, requiring more intensive and expensive care. But how was he going to supply it? He'd already reduced his personnel by 30. And now 12 more positions were on the block.

External forces beyond *his* control were making decisions which affected how *he* functioned, too.

Discouraged and resigned, neither the nurse nor the administrator knew of any alternatives. They had given up hope of ever restoring a sense of control over their lives, of increasing their satisfaction in the jobs they had to perform. They had stopped looking for ways.

But ways *do* exist.

Change at the System Level

These are difficult and uncertain times. There are no simple solutions to the complex problems that affect those in the health care field. But there is a simple program that helps individuals up and down the line feel their autonomy and increase their personal satisfaction. Since the program costs the hospital so little, yet if successful brings them so much, administrators should seriously consider introducing it at the system level—primarily for the good of their patients, but secondarily for the good of their institution.

Hospitals today are looking for ways to be more "customer-sensitive"—or to use the current buzz word, to be "patient-driven." They know that those that come up with a better way will thrive, just as businesses thrive when they launch a better product—one that customers (read patients) instinctively respond to.

I would urge this administrator to take the concept of care partnering directly to his board—armed with actuarial statistics. Insurance companies across the country are discovering what should have been obvious from the start: that when the level of "caring" goes up in hospitals, the number of malpractice suits goes down. According to these statistics, the more sensitive hospitals are to the psychological and emotional needs of patients, families and staff, the lower the stress, the risks and the claims. Some are acting on these statistics. St. Paul Fire and Marine Insurance Company, one of the largest of these companies, insuring over 2,000 hospitals nationwide, is urging its hospital clients to redefine their operations so that patients, families and staff feel more valued, cared for and helped.

Care partnering provides a structure for this "caring." For one thing, it limits the names, faces and services to be remembered and understood. In doing so, it reduces the hospital experience for patients and families, even for staff, to manageable proportions. As modest as that achievement may seem, it's significant. In this era when hospitals merge into giant consortiums and nursing homes are managed by nationwide corporations, any measure that counteracts the impersonal effect of "bigness" can offer a way for an institution to stand out. It will develop a reputation as "a hospital that cares." Its administrators become known as progressive leaders, operating on the leading edge of contemporary health care services.

What's more, the process feeds on itself. Such a reputation attracts forward-looking patients, physicians, staff and insurance carriers. They, in turn, solidify and expand the financial base. As the fortunes of the hospital move up, its successes multiply in a continuously self-reinforcing cycle.

Dr. Peter Koestenbaum, a philosopher who consults with some of our country's largest corporations, contends in his book *The Heart of Business* that if businesses act from the heart, the by-product is almost always increased profits. By the same token, if hospitals return the patient to the center of the health care system and insist that high technology serve rather than dictate human values, financial stability will follow as a matter of course. Care partnering *is* good business.

Change at the Staff Level

But in the absence of a change in the system, a nurse may have to make his or her own changes—simple ones that can be carried out at the staff level. If I were working with Evelyn, I would ask her how she would change her role as a nurse if she could. Guided by her answer, I would show how a care partner program could be confined to whatever elements of nursing were important to her, administered on a case-by-case basis. In many cases, there's no need to change the whole hospital system.

For instance, if we were to set up a care partner program with Evelyn and the McGuires, she could choose how she wished to participate. Could she be assigned to John McGuire each day? Or could she simply drop by between shifts? Maybe she could serve as his advocate during nursing rounds? Why not try?

Change at a Unit Level

Many nurses feel more comfortable with change when they unite with others on their unit. At Planetree, the nurses, like Evelyn, no longer felt right about rotating from patient to patient. They wanted to change their scheduling system so they could be assigned to one patient until that patient was discharged. But the rest of the hospital was on a different plan; and administration didn't know how to schedule one unit differently from the rest. But that didn't stop these nurses. They formed a committee with the administrators; and together they found a plan that worked. The Planetree nurses would only be assigned to the Planetree unit itself and not to other units on the floor. Such a change created the necessary staff stability for primary nursing to begin.

Each time a problem arose, they dealt with it creatively. Instead of reverting to the old system, they just worked with the flaws in the new one. When the pitfalls of primary nursing became apparent (for instance, a difficult patient taxing the endurance of a single nurse), they turned to the basic elements of care partnering described throughout this book—creativity, honesty and choice. No law said that a primary nurse *had* to remain with a long-term patient throughout his stay. No one decreed that a nurse couldn't ask for relief. In the end, they found that nothing they set out to do wasn't fixable, so long as flexibility and a cooperative spirit were present.

Since Planetree's opening, its nurses have taken responsibility for their problems and, therefore, for their solutions. As a unit, they've set their own unit policies. Now, when doctors admit patients to the Planetree unit, they must accept a philosophy that supports patients being informed about their illnesses, families being involved in the care, and nurses being the primary health educators to patients and families.

How have the doctors reacted? Some refuse to admit their patients to the unit. But during Planetree's first year of operation, the number of admitting physicians rose from an original 15 to over 150. And the admitting physicians grew more enthusiastic as time went by. "On the other floors, I can talk to several staff and no one knows exactly what's going on," one physician remarked to me. "On the Planetree unit, I can count on *one* nurse who's willing to be accountable for my patient. I like it more every day."

Can We Give Up Control?

Which brings up the issue of control. Who has it in a hospital? Who's willing to give up some of it and to whom? And what are the rewards for doing so? It's an issue central to the success of the care partner program and critical to all members of its triad—patient, staff member and family. Every patient wants control, writes a Boston psychologist, Dr. Robert Kastenbaum, in an anthologized article appropriately titled "In Control." The physician, the nurse, the therapists, the orderlies want it, too. "It's what janitors want as they mop the floor and hospital administrators as they pick up the telephone . . . Everyone (in the hospital) wants to stay in control."

If Dr. Kastenbaum is right, and this is one of the drives everyone experiences in a hospital, then we must find ways to, at once, use and defuse it. The care partner approach supplies such a way. It encourages all the parties involved to act in ways that enhance their own power—and everyone else's as well. This is crucial. When one party hoards all the control, the environment becomes impoverished. Individuals lose their freedom to create, to give and receive quality care. Everybody loses. Neither the physician nor anyone else in the hospital hierarchy should be allowed to do that to themselves or to anybody else. As Dr. Kastenbaum puts it, nobody should be allowed "to pack all the control into (a) little black bag, and then walk away."

Exercising Positive Control

Here's a list of ways health professionals can experience their power in positive rather than negative ways—in ways that don't compel them to wrest control away from patients and families in order to retain their own.

- *Begin to talk among yourselves.* Set up support and advisory groups for professionals, paraprofessionals and administrative staff. Begin to feel more. Begin to question how things are done.

- *Set up informal care partnering on your own.* Approach a patient and/or family member and start an individual process going.

- *Take some responsibility for change.* Don't hide behind "the system." If you are a member of a system, you're an important cog in its machinery. Your choices can make a difference in how it operates. First, verbalize your feelings. Then act.

- *Show patients how to advocate for professionals who want change.* Patients often have rights and power that you will never have. Teach them how to verbalize their requests, how to use their medical charts, how to request changes in professional behaviors and roles.

- *Limit yourself to only one care partner team at a time. The care partner program should remain special for you. When your energies are focused on one patient who is treated special by you and responds differently to you, the program becomes a welcome change from your standard everyday practice. Conversely, when you must provide care partnering for every person under your care, it may become just another chore.*

- *Look after one another.* Health professionals, like everyone else, need care and attention. Ask for help from
within your ranks. And be prepared to accept help
from whatever source. The POWER OF 3 provides just
that. It offers a unique opportunity for all three of its
elements—patient, family member and professional—
not only to express their needs and expand their options, but to extend care and concern to one another.
Accept it.

Chapter 3

MOVING BEYOND FEAR

The hardest part had been establishing a beachhead. Winning permission from the doctor to sleep in her father's room had been only the first step. Katherine knew the next big hurdle was to get the support of the Coronary Care Unit nurses. The doctor could get her inside, but it would take only one disgruntled nurse to have her removed. She would have to behave in a way that didn't create problems for other families and patients and, most important, for the nursing staff.

Her position was precarious. The first night she slept little. She tried to be inconspicuous. When the nurses came in the room, she contracted her body and held her breath. She didn't dare speak or move from her cot. She didn't even feel safe using the bathroom in her father's room or leaving the CCU for the one down the hall. So all night long she held on. She held her tongue. She held her bladder. She held her position.

Like Katherine, most family members who consider becoming care partners do so with trepidation. They feel ignorant and clumsy around the machinery. They're fearful of doing something wrong. They're afraid of breaking the rules. They're reluctant to speak up, to stand out.

Some never do. They seem incapable of moving beyond visitor status; and to the end, they remain aliens in a foreign land. The majority, however, are fully capable of changing these conditions. Though isolated and full of doubts at the outset, they can grow and become effective in the hospital setting if they can gain control over their fears and move beyond them.

Their first step is to realize that they're not alone, that the "natives" are fearful, too—for different reasons, but with similar consequences. Let's imagine what might have gone on in the minds of the night nurse, the early morning aide and the attending physician when Katherine spent that first 24 hours in her father's room.

> AIDE: . . . *who does she think she is? . . . getting special privileges and all . . . how can I bathe him with her around? . . . can't make a mistake . . . bet she'll go straight to the head nurse.*
>
> NIGHT NURSE: . . . *there's that woman everybody's talking about . . . checking up on me . . . thinks she's got some inside line in here . . .*
>
> DOCTOR: . . . *took notes during evening rounds . . . asked if I'd ordered an EKG . . . what's she doing? . . . collecting evidence . . . just in case?*

A major part of my job in hospitals is to help everyone move beyond debilitating fear. I try to *desensitize* lay people to their fears of illness, hospital machinery, authority figures. With professionals, on the other hand, I try something different. I try to *resensitize* them—put them back in touch with the feelings, instincts and emotions that brought them into the health field in the first place. When nurses, doctors, therapists, technicians are able to reach out to patients as human beings rather than as cases to be treated, the worst fears of hospital staff—financial or administrative repercussions—just never happen. And they often get in touch with their own needs for human love and caring.

This isn't some utopian theory. Those in the business of saving money for hospitals—insurance companies—now recognize this as a fact. And they're beginning to bring pressure on their hospital clients to change how they do this business of "caring." But what insurance companies don't understand is that pressure to change systems will not bring the desired results unless the fears of the individuals involved are first addressed.

WAYS TO DESENSITIZE

In the case of patients and families, the best ways to fight fear of hospitals and what happens in them is, first, to get the facts and, second, to work on attitudes. Fear of pain, disability, institutions, authorities, even death—the most destructive of all fears in hospitals—usually fade, then vanish altogether, when countered by knowledge and a strong, positive outlook.

Knowledge is Power

Nothing banishes fear faster than knowledge. Finding out the facts about hospital routines and procedures, about the illness in question—or anything else related to the problem—defeats the power of the unknown. Planetree offers hundreds of examples of how information can restore confidence and calm. One man who had been diagnosed with lung cancer was so fearful of what that might mean that he wouldn't discuss it, even with his family. But what he *was* willing to discuss—because it didn't seem nearly so threatening to him—was the pacemaker he wore for his weak heart.

So he asked his nurse for a fact sheet about pacemakers, a simple two-page leaflet that explained in laymen's language what pacemakers do, how long they last, and how weak batteries can be detected. When he'd read that information, he asked for more.

The nurse ordered a research packet from the Planetree Resource Center, a bookstore and library for lay people associated with, but separate from, the Planetree hospital unit. This material (over 30 pages of it) finally answered all his questions and gave him a sense of control over his situation. It reduced his anxiety about the cancer by diverting his attention to a problem he was ready to deal with. It gave him time to adjust to the cancer diagnosis. And it showed him how responsive the nurses were to him and his needs. Then, when the time was right—when he felt safe and ready for it—he was able to deal with his cancer.

At Planetree, simple fact sheets about typical diseases, their medications and treatments, are kept right on the ward. When research packets are requested from the Resource Center, they're researched from available sources and, when possible, offered at several reading levels. This way the patient can have access to available information matched to his degree of literacy or interest. After discussion with the patient, the nurse writes up the request to the Resource Center staff, indicating the kinds of questions which need to be answered and the level of sophistication desired. This can range from lay language with lots of drawings, to simple medical language with a few medical illustrations, to detailed medical language with accompanying charts and graphs.

The patient can order packets for care partners as well. One patient due to have corneal transplant surgery ordered a packet for his wife that described how his surgery would take place. It proved invaluable to her. "It gave me something to do," she told me later. "I didn't have to wait around feeling ignorant and helpless. I could follow the operation, step-by-step, from the waiting room."

The Planetree Resource Center pioneered this level of patient education, intended for lay people outside the hospital as well as for those within. Similar facilities now exist in major cities across the United States, some freestanding and some within large medical centers.

For those without access to these specialized libraries, a public library or a hospital medical library may suffice. But often neither will be satisfactory. Your public library may not be equipped to respond to the type of material you request. Your hospital library may be restricted to medical staff only. You may have to bring pressure to bear just to gain access to it. If and when you do, the available material may be too technical to be readily understood.

But more and more patients and families are refusing to tolerate this barrier. They're insisting that hospitals and doctors locate or produce material they *can* understand. And many health professionals are responding. Audio and video tapes are being made available for listening or viewing. Hospital tours are being offered which feature film showings and take-home pamphlets. Question and answer sessions with hospital staff and knowledgeable patients are sometimes included. Following hospital discharge, calls are being made by nurses prepared to respond to queries and concerns.

But what patients want most is an opportunity to talk with their *own doctor*. And they should be able to. Some of the most important advice I give patients and families is this: The word "doctor" comes from the Latin root word *docere*, which means "to teach." If your doctor is not also your teacher, ask him to be. If he declines, find another teacher or another source. In the medical setting, ignorance is not bliss. It is the root of helplessness, dependency and fear. Knowledge is power. *Get it and use it.*

Positive Attitudes/Reinforcing Images

Patients and family members also can combat fear through positive attitudes and images. A patient I once knew worked through his fear of needles by combining knowledge with a change of attitude. Billy, age 40, had been severely beaten in a mugging incident and left for dead. As a result of the multiple operations required to repair his injuries, he'd acquired a phobia of needles. But with the support of a psychologist and an interested lab technician, Billy learned about his veins, the difference between those that were still good and the hard, overused ones. During a procedure, he learned how to assist the technician by holding his arm at the proper angle and by utilizing breathing and relaxation techniques. He handled needles and their containers. And he gave his fear a number on a scale of 1 to 5. In time, by talking about his fear and working with it, he conquered it.

Dr. Viktor Frankl, professor of psychiatry and neurology and author of *Man's Search for Meaning*, calls this a "paradoxical intention," a situation where the fearful person entertains, if only for a moment, that which he or she fears most. To do this, he must be able to see himself once removed. He needs the same detachment that helps him keep his sense of humor in the face of disaster, or when his life seems to be falling apart. By working directly with his fears—even playing with them—he begins to bring them under control.

At the Center for Attitudinal Healing in Tiburon, California, children and adults with life-threatening illnesses come together to teach each other ways to deal with their fears. At one meeting I attended, a woman in her sixties told other cancer patients how she got over her fear of chemotherapy. "I used to dread the pain from the treatment more than the pain from the cancer," she told her support group. "But then I thought, 'Why should I automatically think of treatment as painful? Why can't I associate it with healing?' "

Having entertained that possibility, she set about changing her attitude, then her actions. She wore pretty colors when she went in for treatment. She brought a tape recorder with earphones, and as the chemicals were injected into her body, she listened to her favorite music. She visualized the healing taking place in her cells. In short, by not becoming a victim of the therapy, but rather a participant in it, her fear, and in turn her pain, disappeared.

A child at the center explained how he controlled his pain by use of images. "Every time they stick needles in me," he said, "I think of myself as a marshmallow. Now who can hurt a marshmallow?"

WAYS TO RESENSITIZE

Two nurses entered the room briskly and went over to the bed, checking the IV, then reaching for the folded draw sheet under John's torso.

51

They must have seen Katherine sitting on the folding cot. But they gave no sign of it. One went to one side of John's bed, the second to the other side. Together they reached for the folded sheet, tugged both sides toward the outside, then pulled one side up and over, forcing John's body to roll onto his left side. After adjusting his position with pillows, the second nurse left.

Katherine came around to the remaining nurse. "Whenever you want me to leave during a procedure," she said, "just tell me and I'll go."

The nurse, a taciturn young woman with a thatch of red hair and swarms of freckles over her broad face and strong arms, looked at Katherine with impenetrable blue eyes. Silently, she finished taking John's blood pressure and temperature and put the thermometer back in its case.

Katherine pushed on. "Look, I don't want to be in your way or cause you extra work," she began. "Actually I'm a little scared of you and all the things you do. But I'd like to make myself useful. I know you get short-handed sometimes. If you think it would work, I could learn to help with turning my father over. Then you'd only need to send one person to do it instead of two."

Katherine wasn't sure whether what she'd said had made a difference. She sensed that her awkwardness was touching a responsive chord somewhere behind that impassive gaze.

But she couldn't tell for sure.

Lay people are usually quick to recognize their fears in the hospital setting and are receptive to receiving help when it's offered. Health professionals rarely are. Partly that's because of the expectations laid on them. They're expected to manage any fears they may have of illness and institutions. They expect it of themselves. They expect it of their colleagues. After all, they've been trained in this work.

Their stoicism also stems from the nature of their job. They're expected to maintain the balance between life and death on a daily basis. Constantly on the alert for danger, intent on maintaining their professionalism, they tend to distance themselves from those they care for. And in the process, they often lose their ability to experience normal human emotions. While many have an unexpressed yearning to reverse this, most get more and more out of touch with the caring instincts that might bring it about.

What's worse, they receive little understanding from others for their plight. Katherine had an inkling of the truth. She sensed the right approach to take. But most patients and family members rarely recognize that the abrupt or aloof treatment they often get from doctors and other staff may simply be the masking of fright. Apprehension about making mistakes, uneasiness over deviating from standard practice, suspicion of assertive patients and family members and, most of all, terror about the prospects of potential lawsuits loom heavily over most health professionals. And so the gulf between them and others widens.

However, suggesting to professionals that they are unresponsive to those they're supposed to be serving is usually counterproductive. When confronted with a direct statement of blame, they understandably become defensive. So an indirect approach is usually best. If you expect them to extend care and attention to others, care and attention must first be extended to them.

Care and Attention at the System Level

Care and attention can take many forms. Progressive hospital administrators are beginning to look at how their staff is being treated. At Planetree, unit meetings are held monthly for staff to air complaints. The project administrator attends every meeting and knows each staff person by name. An advisory committee of doctors and nurses meets *jointly* to give advice on unit policy. Staff is given the opportunity to meet weekly with a psychiatric nurse consultant to discuss different approaches to working with difficult patients or personnel. The nursing coordinator is available at any time to discuss these problems. When there are individual problems, she brings individuals together. When there are shift problems, she brings shifts together.

Those are the more orthodox ways of caring for staff. There are some unorthodox ways that are equally effective. Six days a week massage therapists come to the Planetree unit to offer shoulder and neck massages to staff as well as patients. Once a year a staff retreat is held outside the hospital walls. But perhaps more effective than anything are some simple pieces of paper that read, "The Planetree Certificate of Appreciation." These awards can be made by any member of the unit to anyone who has rendered outstanding service, from the neurological consultant to the book chart volunteer.

Overall, what is communicated is this: Staff's needs are taken seriously and staff's ideas, once heard, can lead to action.

Care and Attention at the Heart Level

But the primary place where resensitization occurs is at the heart level. An ordinary person operating at this level can do more than any administrator writing memos or sending out directives.

Take the pediatric units. Here family members first won the right to be regularly involved in their loved ones' care. Here staff have historically been more lenient about hospital rules. Here greater weight has been given to the comfort and pleasure of the patient—whether that has meant putting the nurses in soft pastel colors or bringing in clowns to do magic tricks. One needs only to hear the delighted whispers of an intensive care nurse who has successfully slipped a favorite puppy to a special child to know that this is true. The joy radiated from the experience comes not just from the child, but from every staff member who holds the secret. What this means, then, is this: The key to achieving resensitization lies in the ability of patients and families to touch the hearts of doctors, nurses, aides, technicians—in fact, any member or group of members of the vast hospital team.

7:00 A.M. Half asleep on her hard little cot, Katherine suddenly came to attention. A lab technician had entered the room calling out, "Mr. McGuire, I've come to take a blood sample." Katherine was elated. Someone on staff had finally spoken directly to him, using his name.

But it soon became clear what had happened. The technician hadn't known John was in a coma. When it dawned on her, she glanced at his still body, then at Katherine, and flushed with embarrassment, not knowing what to do next.

"Thanks for calling Dad by name," Katherine said. "Do you mind telling him about this blood test?"

The technician hesitated, looking like she might run from the room. But then in a small voice, gaining volume as she went along, she crossed the line from fear to confidence: "Mr. McGuire, I'm going to take some blood . . ."

Later that day Katherine took out a sheet of butcher paper and a blue felt pen and wrote in large block letters:

"WE CAN'T BE SURE JOHN CAN'T HEAR, SO WE'RE ASSUMING HE MAY BE ABLE TO AND JUST CAN'T

RESPOND. WE TALK TO HIM, READ TO HIM, STROKE AND
PAT HIM. THESE ARE THINGS YOU CAN DO, TOO, IF YOU
FEEL COMFORTABLE WITH THEM."

It doesn't take a pediatric unit and nurses in pastel uniforms for change to take place in a hospital. All it takes is for
people to communicate from the heart. A poster is one way.
At Planetree, they have others—for instance, writing in the
medical chart. In fact, any patient in any hospital can ask to
do this. Direct access may be denied. But if it is, a request can
be made for the next best thing—that written statements be
added to the chart.

Another avenue of communication at Planetree is through
doctors' rounds and patient conferences. This is unusual.
Almost nowhere except in innovative programs like Planetree's, or where exceptional patients or family members have
initiated it, are patients and family members included in
meetings where their treatment is being discussed. Yet, when
you think about it, what could be more fitting? I would, in
fact, go further. I would arrange meetings where patients, in
addition to learning from the experts, would *teach* the experts
by supplying information about their care.

Even more needed is a way to communicate at a deeper
level. The primary task of a care partner facilitator is to get
people to talk to one another about feelings. But sometimes
it's really hard to talk about the deepest levels of our being.
Sometimes unconventional means are needed. For instance, if
people can't say how they feel, they can write letters. Or,
again, they can use the poster approach. They can put a large
sign on a hospital wall that expresses their feelings. One
family wrote this:

"WE APPRECIATE YOUR CARE AND CONCERN FOR ALL
OF US. LET US KNOW HOW WE CAN THANK YOU."

The response they got was overwhelming. But what if they had written this:

"WE'RE REALLY SCARED, AND WE DON'T KNOW HOW TO TELL YOU."

Would they have embarrassed and offended a nurse or social worker unprepared for this kind of revelation? I think not. I've found something happens to staff when patients dare to be emotionally vulnerable, when family members have the courage to reveal their pain and inadequacies. This, in fact, is what sparks the resensitization process. It is more powerful than in-service training, psychiatric consultation, or any book or lecture on the subject.

And patients are in the most strategic position to set it in motion. Illness provides a unique opportunity to experience and express vulnerability. "Once I went public with my pain, it was easy," Harold, an AIDS patient, once told me. He started by confronting his first nurse. "I felt her pulling away from me, like I was going to give her my disease. So I told her how I felt. How alone I was. How scared. That more than anything I needed her to listen, that I needed her to care." By continuing to share his feelings, by unabashedly removing his shields, Harold found ways to reach those around him. Each day he asked directly for what he needed; and each day what he needed came to him.

The effect Harold had on the nursing staff was dramatic. "I was about to leave nursing," one of the staff told me. "But Harold, in some strange way that I don't fully understand, made me into the nurse I always wanted to be." The principle at work here is clear. When people say honestly how much they hurt, more often than not others respond with love. They open up when in the past they've closed down. They say "yes" when in other instances they've said "no." Paradoxically, Harold's strength was in his willingness to show his weakness.

THE FEAR OF LOOKING FOOLISH

Hatha yoga had taught Katherine the importance of the conscious breath. "When we work with the breath," her instructor had said, "we can change the contractions and expansions of the brain. The breath stimulates and relaxes the brain at the same time—and in so doing, it allows the individual to alter consciousness."

This seemed important to her now. She wanted to try directing her father's breath. She didn't really know how. Wasn't sure if it would work. But there was nothing to lose, she decided, except her reputation in Madison County Hospital. If staff came in the room, she could look pretty foolish—teaching breathing to someone in a coma.

Well, she'd just be quiet about it. She drew in her breath slowly and evenly and began coaching her father softly, loud enough for him to hear if he could, but low enough not to draw the attention of the nursing staff. "Breathe in, breathe out. Now steady on the inhale ... That's it, you're getting it now ..."

While patients and family are capable of great resourcefulness and courage in talking about and licking their fears of pain, inadequacy, technology, death, they often stumble over the least justifiable fear of all—the fear that an attitude or act of theirs will be regarded as foolish by others. Most often they worry about the disapproval of important authority figures. And of all the possible fears, this is the one most successful at holding people captive to a dehumanizing hospital system.

Patients can become thoroughly educated on their medical procedures, its risks and its side effects. But when it comes to asking for something unorthodox, such as a care partner program, they can easily lapse into passivity. They're too intimidated by the medical staff to ask for it. Fearing criticism, contempt or, worst of all, rejection by the authority figure in charge, they remain helpless and dependent in a system that refuses to support their chosen form of healing.

When I asked staff in one hospital why they felt the care partner program wouldn't work in their institution, one nurse replied. "Most patients do just as they're told. They ask no questions, make no demands, just like good little boys and girls."

On the other hand, when patients find the courage to ask for and get what they want, whether it be care partnering or something else, they usually find they can have it both ways—the program they've chosen *and* the respect and cooperation of staff. The thing to understand is that the staff is not the enemy. The enemy is the fear of rejection. Everybody likes to be liked. But a pat on the head from the doctor isn't essential. Popularity with the nurses isn't crucial. To carry out a care program, all that is needed is institutional clearance. Once that simple truth is recognized, disapproval can be put in perspective. Rejection can cease to be an issue. And staff acceptance will usually follow.

FEAR OF LOSING FACE

Doctors, nurses, therapists, anyone who works in a hospital setting has the same fear of looking foolish. But to them, the risks appear even greater. Looking foolish, they believe, will inevitably lead to losing face.

"What we'd like is for everyone—all the staff, you, every-body—to talk directly to Dad as if he were completely aware and could understand everything."

Dr. Lloyd heard her say it, but he couldn't quite believe it. There she was standing in the door of her father's room, asking for something totally out of line. Her presumptuousness sometimes amazed him.

But he had to hand it to her. A small woman in her early 40's, she had a passionate energy about her that made him uneasy. She and her sister-in-law had shown a fierce loyalty to their father. A part of him wished that all his patients had relatives who would go to bat for them like that. On the other hand, she was a damned nuisance.

"It'll be no reflection on you—on your professional judgment," she was saying. *"Just write in his chart that the family requests it."*

As he weighed his options, he sized her up. She stood her ground, looking him straight in the eye. He stared back, strangely attracted to her idea, but stopped by a ground swell of resistance welling up from deep inside him.

While I was having dinner recently with a doctor and his wife, I asked him why his colleagues in such situations find it harder than other people to grant a request like that. He said it was due to their greater objectivity. But his wife knew better. Intuitively grasping what he failed to note she said, "They're more afraid of looking foolish."

I've found that if this fear isn't addressed directly with health professionals, the chances are slim that anyone's behavior will change. But if fear is faced squarely, it can often be overcome. It eventually was in Katherine's case. Katherine had guessed that the real obstacle to the doctor's speaking directly to her father was the doctor's fear of losing face in the eyes of his colleagues. She also sensed he was unlikely to change unless she could convince him that writing this instruction in her father's chart wouldn't make *him* look bad. If she could give him a way to ascribe his actions to the wishes of the family, she knew she would be able to sway him.

The fear of losing face imposes severe limitations on all staff. It particularly afflicts newly graduated nurses, beginning interns and residents, or anyone whose hospital reputation is not secure. But those willing to confront and conquer it can find the effort more than worthwhile. They find themselves emancipated. They are free at last to transcend the restrictions of typical hospital life, ready to challenge the old and to sample and benefit from the new.

THE FOOL: THE SUPREME ADVENTURER

The fool is both the lowest and the highest card in the Tarot deck, a set of cards used for centuries by sages to predict the future and understand the present and the past. On the face of the fool's card is a youth holding a white rose while stepping fearlessly off a cliff. The fool, we are told, symbolizes the life-breath, the supreme adventurer passing through the gates of experience to divine wisdom. Whether or not one accepts the practice of tarot reading, I believe we can learn from the symbolism embodied in its cards. Until we can feel confident enough in ourselves to be judged a fool by others, we cannot be fully free to express ourselves, much less to adventure beyond what is already known or accepted.

LOOKING FEAR IN THE EYE

Throughout this chapter, I've talked about ways to understand and accept our fears so we can reframe our thoughts and feelings about them. Here are some specific suggestions for action.

- *Gather Your Facts:* Get educated about your fear through every possible source—books, films, articles, tapes, classes, workshops, self-help groups, or any knowledgeable person available to you.

- *Talk About Your Fear:* Talking about fear makes a difference even if we talk only to ourselves. By talking to ourselves or others, we become aware of what our fears really consist of. They are often centered on a worry about the future or an anxiety about losing control. What will happen *if?* What will people think *then?* What will I be like *when?* Note that these questions largely derive from comparing ourselves to others. "I feel I'm not clever enough, articulate enough, attractive enough to do that. Someone else is smarter, wiser, cooler under pressure."

- *Look at Alternatives. Plan Options:* Sometimes our fears come from feeling we have no choices. After you've gathered all your facts, make a list of alternatives to your present situation. And remember, even when your options are limited, you always have a choice of attitude.

- *Monitor Your Emotional Response:* Rate your fears and give them numerical values. "Look out, here comes a big #5. Only a #2? No problem, I can handle that." When you label your fears, you can play with them, possibly even laugh at them.

- *Use Positive Imagery and Visualizations:* Think through a hospital situation that would frighten you most. Visualize an experience that might prepare you for that fear. Figure out what you would want your family, friends or colleagues to do or not do for you in such an emergency. You can be very practical in this exercise or very fanciful.

  Now picture the place, the people, the circumstances clearly in your mind. See your family, friends, colleagues there offering you support. Feel this support throughout your body. See the hospital staff accepting you and your ideas. Create an active image of yourself surmounting your worst fear, an image which pictures you literally clearing a physical hurdle and sailing to a successful landing on the other side.

- *Breathe:* The quickest and best method of stress reduction is deep breathing. Begin by exhaling fully. Then inhale, letting the abdomen expand as if you were filling a balloon with air. Let the lower chest expand, allowing the rib cage to expand, then the upper chest all the way to the collar bones. On the exhalation, let the upper chest contract, the middle chest, then the abdomen, pulling the abdomen toward the spine. Continue in a rhythmic and comfortable fashion.

  This is an exercise that can be done to prepare for surgery. It can be done by family members waiting for the results. And it can be done by the operating room team as the surgery is performed. You'll find when you are breathing deeply, it's virtually impossible to hold onto anxiety and fear. You are taking as much as seven times more oxygen than you normally do, and it is going to all parts of your body, including the brain. Your body and your mind are immediately calmed.

- *Move Your Body:* To deal concretely with fear, try simple physical movement. Any movement will do. Patients should ask their doctors or their physical therapists what stretching exercises (range of motion) they can do in bed. Family members should try walking in the hospital hallways or around the grounds. Some simple yoga stretches can be done unobtrusively right in the hospital room.

- *Get Tough with the Little Fears:* Begin to practice on the little fears. Small timidities can lead to big retreats, especially in hospitals. Begin to notice the little capitulations that multiply in the routines of hospital life. Will you ask for another pitcher of ice water? Will you speak to your supervisor about something important to you? Will you introduce yourself to another family member on the ward? Begin doing battle with these chronic fears, the little ones that lower self-esteem. By proving yourself on this battleground, you will develop more faith in your capacity to handle major stresses.

- *Show Your Power Through Your Love:* When your power comes from an assertion of love, it can actually rid you of your fears. Check your posture. Stand or sit erect. Open your chest, breathe deeply, and use space as you walk, stand or sit. This practice actually raises your confidence level. Can you imagine a samurai warrior moving around the battlefield like most of us cower around the hospital?

  Now with your chest spread fully, imagine your heart opening up to others. What I am suggesting is actually an amalgam of assertiveness and love—ordinary people like you and me moving with the poise and self-confidence of warriors. But rather than acting in anger, we are sending forth a powerful current of love to everyone we meet. If you can't relate to the samurai warrior approach, use your own personal imagery or some caring action you choose to perform for someone in your midst. What you'll find is you can't hold on to fear and give forth love at the same time.

- *Befriend Your Fear:* Begin to take the "fangs" out of fear. "Oh, hello, fear. I remember you. The last time you came to see me was when I told my doctor I was seeking a second opinion."

  This process of making friends with fear is helped if you can consider the *positive* things fear does for you. Here's a list I began once:

  1. Fear raises my adrenalin level, gives me more energy and moves me into action.
  2. Fear increases my excitement level and wards off boredom.
  3. Fear teaches me humility.
  4. Fear allows me to test my courage and my strength.
  5. Fear opens up avenues for spiritual development.
  6. Fear protects me from dangers that threaten me.

- *Recognize Your Need for Fear:* I appreciate my fear most for taking care of me, protecting me from situations I feel I'm not yet ready to accept. In other words, occasionally we *need* our fear. Some of us permit help from others only when we're frightened and helpless. In medical situations we may all need to be taken care of by others, if only for short periods. And this is where fear can temporarily become our friend. It allows us to receive such help. It makes it O.K. to be

65

nurtured. What's more, it's a process which builds on itself. A nourished person is a person better able to give to others, and a person able to give is a person able to transcend fear.

What all this ultimately points to is this: After recognizing, labeling and, when appropriate, placing a positive value on our fears, we usually find we can let go of them. And once we've let go of fear, we discover almost anything is possible. If we peel back the outer layers of our most painful emotions—anger, guilt, anxiety, depression—we usually find at their core the primitive emotion of fear. It follows, then, that if patients, family members and professionals can liberate themselves from fear, they can break out of the prison of their personal restraints and walk in the open. When that happens, they are ready to build successful relationships, and through them effective care partnerships.

Chapter 4

STRENGTHENING THE CARE PARTNERSHIP

The doctor and Katherine were about to begin one of their hall-way rituals. He leaning against the wall, his arms hugging his crisp white chest, one shoulder lifted defensively. She, circling around him, keeping her distance, starting with an open-ended question and hoping it would lead them somewhere.

"We realize that Dad's condition is very serious," she began, letting him know that she had faced and accepted the truth. "Is there something the family needs to know now? So we can decide what to do?"

He looked down at his watch, turned his body away from her and murmured something she couldn't make out. Was he really too busy right now? Or just too anxious to answer her? She couldn't tell. But the subject was too important to drop. She changed her position, established eye contact, and tried again. "Are we going to have to make a decision about keeping him alive?"

"Let's wait and see," he said, indicating by his tone that he had nothing more to say. She paused for a moment, wondering how to

penetrate his wall of silence. But before she could speak, he'd disappeared into the next room.

In a care partnership that is functioning well, all parties to it will enjoy a feeling of mutual trust and respect. Each will experience the confidence that comes from working as an equal member of a health care team.

When this doesn't happen, it's usually because one party has slipped back into the one/up—one/down pattern traditionally true of medical interactions. Regressions like this can be brought on by the professional care partner or by a professional outside the triad. Most often it involves a physician. But no matter who is responsible, the root cause is almost always an imbalance of power. And the solution lies in each member of the partnership becoming aware of how he or she has contributed to it.

AN IMBALANCE OF POWER

He began his daily report. "Blood chemistries good. Temperature normal yesterday, beginning to drift up today. Maybe something more definitive tomorrow." He turned and started down the hall. Katherine was at his heels, this time determined to get an answer.

Just short of the elevator, she got her answer. Wheeling around and confronting her, he blurted out his exasperation. "Look, Mrs. Hogan, I have other patients in this hospital. At this time, I have nothing else to tell you."

The elevator doors had opened and he was backing through them. As he pressed the "Up" button, and his escape route became assured, his voice took on a conciliatory tone. Calling out to the solitary figure in the hallway, he asked,"Have you thought of going back to California?"

As he spoke, the elevator doors, sliding noiselessly along their tracks, closed in front of him, touching together with a clean, decisive bang. A second later, he was up and away.

In this situation, an impasse was inevitable. The doctor had near total control over the time and place of the meeting. He had inside information about the rules of the game. He could manipulate the terms of the negotiations. And so he did.

In these circumstances, *most* doctors do. In fact, nurses, social workers, therapists, technicians—everyone up and down the hospital hierarchy—can easily revert to seizing power and control. When, under such conditions, they're challenged about their behavior, they'll say that they do it to save time. But for many it's a long established tradition, hardened into a rigid and insensitive habit.

For some it may have even deeper roots. Dr. Paul Brenner, a California physician and lecturer, has been honest enough to say in workshops he conducts for health professionals around the country, "It was a rude awakening when I first realized that I needed patients to be sick and dependent on me, so I, Paul Brenner, could feel good about myself."

If such a problem arises among care partners, they should look again at their agreement. The agreement should define the rights of all sides and provide the negotiating tools for eliminating inequities. It should also provide the opportunity for all parties to become more aware of personal needs.

When the problem lies outside the triad, which is often the case, the professional on the team can serve as an impartial observer, commenting on behaviors that seem to be contributing to the impasse, and supporting other people's actions to correct it. Or this person can adopt a more direct problem-solving role, as either a facilitator or an arbitrator, actively helping the parties change the dynamics of their interactions.

Because when even *one* person changes his or her behavior, the dynamics *do* change. Though patients and families sometimes don't believe it, no one can have power over them unless they, at some level, choose to give their own power away.

The care partner approach is intended to make all parties more aware of their attitudes and how they affect the way power is dispersed. The care partner agreement is a means of spreading the power around: by assigning equal responsibilities, conferring equal benefits, awarding equal rewards for work well done. Through its application, patients and family members learn how to gain power directly without manipulation or one-upmanship. And professionals learn the rewards of voluntarily sharing power. Through this process all parties work together as adults rather than in the unconscious ways of the past.

HOW EVERYONE CAN WIN

Most people think the only way to gain power is to take it away from others. But there's a more effective way. *Give* power to yourself. Throughout this book, I offer some ideas for reducing fear by placing a greater value on ourselves—from issuing ultimatums to our mirror to striding through hospital corridors as benevolent samurai warriors. This same principle works for strengthening lay/professional partnerships. In the medical setting the best way to effect this shift is to relinquish our comfortable dependence on doctors and nurses, our need to see them as parent figures.

"Whether they realize it or not, many of my patients turn childlike the moment they walk through my door," says one doctor I know. "It's as if they're looking to me for rewards and punishment." His experience is all too common. In the presence of a doctor, many of us who function quite normally in other areas of our lives will revert to the child within—the child still yearning for the love and approval of a long ago parent.

"Captains of industry who chop off heads without batting an eye walk into hospitals like infants," says Lowell Levin, Professor of Public Health at Yale School of Medicine. Individuals with enormous clout in other areas of their lives cower at the sight of a white coat. Small wonder, then, that they're treated accordingly.

However these relationships *can* be based on equality and mutual respect. And since, initially at least, patients and family members have the most to gain, they must usually take the first step. This chapter helps them do that. While on the surface the material may seem chiefly concerned with advancing the interests of patients and families, by chapter's end it will become clear that if patients and families can become winners, *everybody* in the health care system wins as well. In a hospital in which personal autonomy, mutual respect and a sense of control are fostered, there are no losers. Secondary payoffs may be different in each case, but the ultimate reward is the same for everyone: physical and emotional wellness, not only for the individuals involved, but for the institution as well.

THE REWARD

For the Patient, It's Getting Well

In the case of the patient, the beneficial effects of having one's autonomy honored—and the damaging effects of this not happening—are apparent from the very beginning of life. Dr. Frederick LeBoyer, author of *Birth Without Violence*, says this: "Most people don't talk to newborn babies. The baby is checked as one checks a machine, rather than as somebody who is very aware of what is going on and is terrified and, moreover, infuriated and humiliated not to be understood as already being somebody . . . The baby is trying to make people understand. It doesn't talk, of course, but it's expressing that it doesn't very much like the way it's being treated. It is suffering in its heart, not in its body, infuriated not to be understood for what it is."

Of course, at any age we feel better when we are treated with dignity and respect, but does it really improve our physical health? Dr. James Fries and Dr. Lawrence Crapo, physicians and joint authors of *Vitality and Aging*, point to numerous studies done around the world showing a positive correlation between health and well-being and the degree of autonomy and control an individual has over his or her environment.

At Planetree, we've made similar findings. As mentioned earlier, a kitchenette was placed on the unit so family members could prepare food for their loved ones. What was not anticipated was that patients would walk into it and start cooking for themselves. The moment the staff stopped treating the patients as if they were helpless, they started behaving as if they were well.

Aggression and assertion can play a role, too. A study by the University of California in San Francisco and the State University of New York in Albany of 639 elderly men and women in institutions and state hospitals demonstrated that overly cheerful and cooperative patients die faster than their more aggressive and "difficult" contemporaries. Asked what survival tips he would give his grandmother, the researcher replied without hesitation, "Show more aggression and stand up for [your] rights."

For the Family, It's Staying Well

When family members submit to hospital rules and procedures that don't feel right to them, they often sustain subtle, but long-term damage to their emotional, if not their physical health. When I began working on this book, several people were referred to me who, earlier in their lives, had been required to make life-support decisions for loved ones. And what I found was that most persons who had been rushed through this process, no matter what the final decision or its outcome, endured years of guilt and remorse. Or they had feelings of anger directed towards themselves or another family member.

That fact is tragic enough in itself. But what makes it doubly poignant is that if these families had been listened to—if they had been allowed to participate more fully in the care of their loved ones—most or all of this bitter aftermath could have been avoided. Dr. Elisabeth Kübler-Ross, a noted expert in the field of death and dying, says when families have ways to externalize their pain through caregiving, they can be free of guilt, fear and shame.

Mary Catherine Bateson, anthropologist and daughter of anthropologists Gregory Bateson and Margaret Mead, added confirmation in her description of her attendance during her father's death: "The shadows of guilt and anger which so often complicate grief may be related to interruptions in the process of caring, and they may be lightened by the experience of tending someone we love with our own hands, so that much that seems externally repellent and painful is transmuted by tenderness."

For Health Professionals, It's Restoring Personal Wellness

Stress and pressure are an inevitable part of the professional lives of hospital workers. Some thrive on it. Others are drained physically and emotionally. Some never recover. Under present conditions, the hazards and health risks for professionals are extreme.

The nurse is sometimes described as a soldier in a combat zone—continually surrounded by blood, vomitus, excreta, exposed genitalia and mutilated bodies. Besides the psychological deadening that occurs in the profession, nurses and others doing direct patient care are at risk of, among other things, muscle strain, cuts, radiation, infection and, now with the AIDS crisis, even death. When an error can be life threatening, every move carries the potential for dire consequences.

In addition to the physical threats, there are the psychological ones. Nurses live in an environment of chronic overstimulation little recognized by patients, administrators or even doctors. Moreover, they often see themselves in an untenable position—assigned an awesome responsibility, but given little authority to act.

Doctors have the opposite problem. For the most part, they hold the power. Accordingly, they are held ultimately accountable for the outcomes, good and bad. The high incidence of alcoholism, drug addiction, suicide and early death in this profession says something about the lives they must lead.

But professionals often create their own stress factors. Holding on to power is a major way to create and maintain stress. Power struggles lead to the kind of brusque professionalism which undermines the very qualities of sensitivity and caring important to healing and to ultimate job satisfaction.

On the other hand, sharing control with patients and family members means sharing responsibility with them as well. Too much control leads to stress and "burn-out," and eventually to illness. Shared control means shared responsibility, lessening the stress on one person and spreading it around to many.

The care partner experiment at Planetree and other hospitals has amply demonstrated this. When lay people are involved in the health care of people they love, not only do they and their patients experience heightened levels of satisfaction and self-esteem, they also reduce, in a very immediate and practical way, the work load of the staff.

This often leads to care partnering's most important bonus for professionals—the capacity to raise their self-esteem and morale. A physical therapist made this observation following a care partner experience in a nursing home. "What I appreciated most from the family was their participation, their interest. It revitalized my interest. . . . Their caring filtered down to the staff and we wanted to give the patient even more attention. It wasn't that we had to anymore. It had more to do with how good we felt about ourselves. They raised morale around here like I've never seen before."

For Hospital Administrators,
It's Institutional Wellness

Read any journal written for health care executives and you see articles with titles like this: "Toward the Patient-Driven Hospital," "The Economics of Patient Satisfaction," "Developing a Consumer-Driven Hospital," "What Do Consumers Really Want?" "Creating the Responsive Organization." On studying the articles closer, you'll see that management experts across the country are strongly recommending that hospital administrators give better customer service by treating patients with more respect and giving them more autonomy. They believe this is the business strategy needed to give individual hospitals the competitive edge they require to survive. Those administrators interested in what's good for patients and families are learning fast that this translates into institutional wellness, even institutional survival.

BEGINNING THE RESHUFFLE

So when one party is holding all the cards, everyone suffers, including the card holder. But why must the hospital game be played by such rules? With the POWER OF 3, we can reshuffle the deck. When we all assume greater power, by definition we place greater value on ourselves. As we feel our value, we abandon immature behaviors toward one another. And as we shed these behaviors, we cause others to abandon their immature behaviors toward us.

To begin the reshuffle, here are some things that patients and families should know.

KNOWING YOUR RIGHTS

"Wish we'd found this sooner," Sarah said after glancing at the first paragraph. The "Patient's Bill of Rights" lay spread out on the bed, a document they'd stumbled onto almost by accident, while visiting the social service office.

"Look here, this is what we're after: Number One. The patient has the right to considerate and respectful care. Number Two. The

patient has the right to obtain from his physician complete current information concerning his diagnosis, treatment, and prognosis in terms the patient can be reasonably expected to understand . . ."

"So we're not that radical after all," Sarah laughed. "Let's write this in ordinary words. Maybe in a letter."

And with that, Sarah and Katherine began the first of a series of letters they would send to the Madison County Hospital staff in the coming days . . .

> "Dear Staff,
>
> In our way, we are trying to do our best for John McGuire. The family wants to work with you to accomplish these goals. Here are some things that are important to us.
>
> We want everyone to approach John just as if he were fully alert and could hear. Tell him what is current about his illness . . ."

All patients have rights, some guaranteed by law and others, as in the "Patient's Bill of Rights," recommended and endorsed by professional associations. These rights give us crucial leverage with persons in power and help us monitor the quality of our care. But most important, they remind us that we're entitled to be treated with dignity and respect.

They guide professionals as well. The "Patient's Bill of Rights" and the "Patient's Rights in a Nursing Home" join the Hippocratic Oath and other professional codes of ethics in supporting nurses, social workers, physicians and others who truly want to keep their professional standards high.

Many people have no idea of their rights in a hospital or nursing home and how they can protect them. On the following pages is a brief sampling of legal and moral rights in health care settings and how I interpret them.

- *Informed Consent:* Physicians are required by law to get a patient's "informed consent" before they administer any treatment. That means they're supposed to fully outline all the options available and the benefits and risks involved in each; and before proceeding, they're supposed to get the patient's permission.

  If you're a patient and don't want to know the risks of treatment, you have a right *not* to know. But it's up to you to let the doctor know your wishes. Some patients function best with a lot of information at their disposal. Others prefer to leave the details to their doctors. But the doctor can't be expected to tell one from the other. So take the responsibility to make that distinction and specify how much information is desired, what kind, and in what form. Without *explicit* instructions to the doctor, you place yourself in a passive role, asking your doctor not only to be your mind reader, but in most cases your decision maker. If that happens—and if the resulting decision goes against your wishes—then you have only yourself to blame.

- *A Second Opinion:* If you're not satisfied with your doctor's recommendation, ask for a second opinion, a third, or a fourth. Doctors do this when they're in doubt. Why not you?

  But if you avail yourself of this option, you need to know how it may play out. If your doctor feels it's not medically proper to go on with a procedure you've requested, either one of you can request medical consultation from another doctor. If the consultant concurs with your doctor, your doctor will normally present these findings to you. If you persist in going against his advice, he can (and indeed should) withdraw from the case and get someone else to take over.

- *Firing Your Doctor:* Sometimes a doctor's recommendations and choices of treatment are unacceptable to you, but he has *not* offered to withdraw from the case and there is no room for compromise. In that case, you may have to ask him to leave. Patients often hesitate to do this. They'll go through all kinds of expensive and painful procedures before facing up to it. But this is clearly your right. Since *you* have hired *him*, you can certainly *fire* him if you're not satisfied with his work.

  Such an action, however, shouldn't be taken lightly. As in any employer/employee relationship, you need to assess how essential this person is to you and whether there are others who can fill the position. If you decide that there are, and you opt to end the relationship, put it in terms that suggest both sides will be better off if there's a parting of the ways.

- *Against Medical Advice:* Even in situations where the choice of doctors is limited—in certain health maintenance organizations, in military and veteran health services, or in small towns with few practicing physicians—you always have the right to go against medical advice. While it usually entails some risk, this recourse, called "AMA" in official medical records, is always available to you as a last resort.

- *Hospital Consent Forms:* When you're admitted to the hospital, you'll be asked to sign its consent forms. Be sure you read them carefully. What's more, feel free to edit them. I know a patient who, as she was being admitted to have her baby, specified in writing that Scopalamine, the "twilight sleep" drug that produces amnesia in the new mother, should not be administered under any circumstances. Even though she'd

79

discussed this many times with her doctor, she wanted to be sure her instructions were known to *all* hospital personnel, so that nobody could later use the excuse, "Nobody told me." Another patient I know, admitted to a teaching hospital, directed that no resident or intern be substituted for her surgeon after she was under anesthesia.

These people felt compelled to issue special instructions because they knew that hospital consent forms, contracts, arbitration agreements do not necessarily guarantee two-way protection. Just like most business contracts, they are designed and intended for the convenience and protection of the presenting party. It is therefore your privilege, indeed your responsibility, to see that *you*—the other party to the agreement—are protected with your own specially written provisions. Actually, such vigilance is a two-way street. It not only assures you of the level of care you desire and expect, it prevents later disagreements and misunderstandings that can negatively impact the hospital. In the end, a two-way consent form protects both parties.

- *Your Medical Chart:* In most states in this country, you have the right to read what others are writing about you and your illness. And you have the responsibility to make sure that what is said in it is correct. An article in a May 1985 issue of the *Wall Street Journal* told of a patient with lung cancer who found on examining her medical chart that she'd been diagnosed a paranoid schizophrenic. But she was obviously in excellent mental health. When confronted with his mistake, her surgeon pleaded human error. A resident on duty, when making an entry, had misunderstood some of his illegibly written notes.

Getting direct access to your chart will not be easy."Of all things the patient could do to rock the boat, that would be it," Edward Bartlett, a public health professor at the University of Alabama at Birmingham is quoted as saying in the same *Wall Street Journal* article. "It's a sensitive area to hospitals because the chart is the inner sanctum of all the secrets."

Some physicians at Planetree's host hospital, Pacific Presbyterian Medical Center, refuse to admit their patients to the Planetree unit because of its open chart policy. Even in states where there are laws guaranteeing patients access to their charts, health professionals don't give out records lightly. And, when viewed strictly from their point of view, this makes some sense. They feel the data contained there will be misunderstood by patients. They also fear, rightly or wrongly, that such information may actually encourage patients to use the entries against them in malpractice suits.

Nevertheless, whether doctors or nurses like it or not, some degree of access to medical records has been upheld by law in most states in this country; and that right is upheld in principle by the American Medical Association, the American Medical Records Association, and by most court rulings handed down in states where there are no relevant statutes. "In every state, if you sue, you get access," says George Annas, Professor of Health Law at Boston University and author of *The Rights of Hospital Patients*, an American Civil Liberties Union guidebook.

Some doctors see no threat in full disclosure. On the contrary, they see advantages. Dr. Hugh Schade of Los Gatos and San Jose, California, has routinely given out full records, including x-ray and test results and his own observations and prescription orders. "Other doctors warn me against it," he says. "But I feel it educates my patients and helps me into the bargain. They read the record, they ask questions, and they learn. They take responsibility for what's in the records, and in the process they take responsibility for their own health."

At Planetree, the staff recommends that patients take advantage of the opportunity to write in their charts. Granted, patients don't always respond. Many feel they have nothing important to say. But, in fact, their day-to-day perceptions of their progress are often far more useful than any nurse's or doctor's interpretation of that experience. In hospitals where there is no open chart policy, I suggest that patients write letters or diary entries to be added to their charts.

Some of us are sympathetic to both sides of the open chart controversy. We can understand doctors' reluctance to make charts available. For one thing, many people, staff as well as patients, have trouble deciphering the abbreviations, medical jargon, and hasty scribbles typically found in most charts. For another, many patients don't want to know the details of their illness and would be adversely affected if they did. These people have a simple recourse, however. They can simply not seek out their chart. And if it is offered by staff, they can refuse to look at it.

If you, on the other hand, are one of those who wants access, and if you live in a state where you have this legal right, don't be deterred. *To read or not to read is your decision to make, not the staff's.* Nothing should stand in the way of your legal right, whether exercised or not, to see both the hospital's records and the doctor's office records. While they own the paper and need not give that up, the facts belong to you. Pay the copying fee and claim what is yours.

- *A Chart of Your Own Creation:* What I wholeheartedly recommend is that you set up your own chart. When I work with care partners, one of my first suggestions is that they buy a notebook and begin making entries. Here they have the right to record, without hassle, anything important to them—temperature and blood pressure, comments by the doctor, names of visitors, stanzas from songs that can be sung in the sick room, words from poems that can be read. The list of possible information is endless. When no family member is present, and the patient is asleep or too ill to preside over entries, the log book can become a register for guests to record their visits and for staff to leave notes. When the family member on day shift hears important information from the doctor or nurse, it can be noted for the family member on the night shift.

Log books are often set up in home care situations. Through them, easily understood information, written in plain English, is passed naturally among everyone on the home care team, including the patient. In these environments, their benefits can't help but be obvious. In hospitals, on the other hand, where staff may not see their value, you may have to take the initiative to begin such a book on your own—and to supply convincing proof of its value.

For staff, a log book can enhance efficiency and increase the quality of the care. By not having to repeat the same information to everyone who enters the scene, nurses and doctors save time and trouble. At the same time, they are assured of a company of well informed lay people, all of whom are up to date on the patient's condition.

As for patients, log books can save lives. A friend of mine and her family started a log following her father's cardiac valve replacement. The nurses had routinely recorded his fluid intake by IV and nasogastric feedings. But after the tubes were removed, the amount of liquids he took by mouth was recorded only in the family record.

As the days went by, the patient's condition began to deteriorate, and he became confused and disoriented. Searching for clues, my friend asked the doctor, "Should he be taking more liquids?" Staff was at a loss to comment. They had no records.

But the doctor agreed to scan the family's log; and it took just one glance for him to hit on the problem. The patient was in an advanced state of dehydration. If the condition had gone on a day or two longer, he would have died. But once it was identified and treated, recovery progressed on schedule.

SPEAKING OUT TO AUTHORITY FIGURES

Katherine slumped into a chair next to Dr. David Gowan, her professional care partner. A few days earlier, after she'd outlined the kind of person she wanted, first to herself, then to Reverend Bingham, the choice of Dr. Gowan had been obvious.

She had asked him to be her friend, not her father's doctor; he'd accepted and their partnership had begun. After he made rounds on his regular patients each morning, he came by to check on Katherine. His support usually required only a few minutes at a time. Sometimes they talked, sometimes they only smiled and waved to one another.

But today, she needed more from him. She needed his advice. She wasn't getting anywhere with Dr. Lloyd. And it was clear she should try another tack. But what?

"I know how much you care about your father. But does Dr. Lloyd know?" Dr. Gowan asked her. "You need to let him know. Tell him how much you need information from him."

"Fine, but how? I'm becoming a pest. Dr. Lloyd runs the other way when he sees me."

"Listen, if a doctor comes in every day and says 'everything's the same' and walks out, you have a right to do something about it." Dr. Gowan leaned forward in his chair and spoke each word slowly and deliberately. "Doctors need to realize that families don't stay at the bedside seven days in a row, 24 hours a day, unless they really care. They aren't there because they don't have any place else to go. At first, it might be a shock to your doctor if you grabbed him by the arm and said, 'I want to talk to you.' But if you did, even once, he wouldn't have to be told twice. You'd have his attention."

Dr. Gowan leaned back in his chair, a faint suggestion of a smile around his mouth, "Don't get me wrong," he said, "I'm not saying you should grab his arm, literally. I'm saying you should grab his attention—by your love, your determination, and the way you express yourself."

Not expressing herself well? How could that be? She'd always been a verbal person—never at a loss for words. Why

85

a breakdown in communication now? The reasons were no doubt complex.

What Katherine didn't realize was that the strategies needed here were of a different order from those that had worked for her in the past. She'd begun with her usual "I-messages." "I feel uninformed," she'd stated directly and clearly. "I need more facts." But even with her best communication skills, she had not been heard. With little or no leverage, seemingly stuck at the lowest rung of the hospital hierarchy, she had to have more than her normal verbal agility. To get Dr. Lloyd's attention, Katherine needed a conscious strategy.

Here are two simple assertive communication techniques which, without anyone becoming loud, angry or obnoxious, can be effective in hospital contexts. In extreme situations, to get a doctor or administrator—or anyone in authority—to stop and listen, use the "broken record" approach. Maintain a calm, noncompetitive tone, but keep speaking, clearly and directly, about what you want. If what you are saying evokes a hostile response, try the technique of "fogging." Visualize your opposition as a fog bank, acknowledge its presence, but politely continue to drive right on through it. Always recognize and try to understand what the other person has to say. If that person makes sense, be willing to change your mind. If not, refuse to be deterred.

Here's an example. The doctor responds to your request to see the results of your lab reports with an evasive tactic. "It's unlikely that you would understand what it means. The policy of the hospital is not to make test results available to the patient, unless there's a special reason to do so." You persist. "I know that's the hospital's standard policy. But patients *do* have a right to see these results if they choose. And I feel it would benefit me to see them."

86

Most people, even authority figures, have only a set number of "no's" in their arsenals. If they tell you "no" six times, ask them seven times. What you are communicating is this: What I want is important to me. I will not be put off. I can do this all day and all night if necessary, even from flat on my back in this bed.

The "broken record" technique can, of course, backfire. If attempted as a power play—if overbearing or insensitive—it can produce results diametrically opposed to those you want. You must let the other person know how important this issue is to you. You must listen attentively and respectfully to him. You must avoid any attempt at intimidation, either through open displays of anger or subtle assignment of guilt. *But you mustn't be deterred from saying what you have to say.*

If you are the patient, and you are too weak or too ill to stand up for yourself, or you simply don't have the temperament for it, get someone else to do it for you. Never find yourself in a hospital without an advocate.

If you are under 18, there will be no problem with your parents speaking for you. But if you are over 18 and deemed legally competent to handle your own affairs, you must make absolutely clear to the staff that you have authorized your advocate to speak for you and act in your interests. Spell it out in writing in your medical chart. Without this clear statement of your intent, your representative is likely to be bypassed. Unless you have given your explicit permission, even a close family member will be prevented from intervening in the professional/patient relationship.

If you can, try to speak for yourself. Granted, it's not easy. Doctors and hospital staff not used to this philosophy of a balance of power may tend to give passive patients subtle psychological rewards (more attention, small kindnesses) for remaining that way. They may hook your guilt through the introduction of minor side issues that put you at a disadvantage. If you become assertive, they may withdraw all rewards and openly reprimand you.

The way to get around this is obvious. At the very outset of the relationship, be clear with yourself that you're not giving anyone authority to confer rewards and punishments. Don't let anyone become parent to your child within. Don't agree to let extraneous issues provoke guilt and contrition. Insist on sticking to the core issues and to your right to be dealt with as an adult.

What you gain can be substantial. Speaking out not only boosts your self-esteem, on rare occasions it can save your life. Doctors can—and do—make mistakes, and the hospital staff can blunder. The People's Medical Society of Emmaus, Pennsylvania, has found that 20% of all those who enter American hospitals develop health complications caused by doctors and/or hospital staff. The most common hazards cited are medication errors, excessive testing and infection. It follows, then, that you should be on constant alert for anything that doesn't feel right to you; and if you note something, that you should speak out. By doing so, you could be preventing a critical illness or even death. According to Dr. Lowell Levin, quoted in the *Wall Street Journal* article reporting these findings, the message is clear: "Don't be a good patient. Be an active patient. Passivity kills."

UNDERSTANDING THE RULES
(AND INTRODUCING SOME OF YOUR OWN)

Dr. Lloyd appeared in the room, keeping well within reach of the door for his usual fast exit. But this time Katherine was ready.

"Please come in," she said, "and sit down." She ushered him to a chair. "We understand you have about ten minutes to give

us—and we promise not to take a minute more. But during that time, we'd like to ask you some questions. I have them written down, so we won't waste any time."

The doctor, poised uncertainly on the edge of the hard plastic seat, seemed at a loss for words. Robbed of the familiar format of his daily "report," he nodded mutely for Katherine to proceed.

So you've begun to make waves: won the staff's attention, signaled doctors, as well as nurses, that you intend to be taken seriously. But this often isn't enough. Somehow you sense there's still a force, generated from within the hospital hierarchy and integral to its operations, working against you, denying you a truly meaningful role in your care program.

In time you discover what powers this all-pervasive force. It's "the rules." Not the rules in the hospital bulletin or those explained to you on admission: No phone calls after 10 P.M. No more than two visitors at a time. "The rules" are more subtle—unwritten, unspoken, and usually unknown to the average patient and family.

Firmly enforced, they often set the tone of relationships between patients, families and professional staff. And those who understand them frequently use them to control these relationships.

Katherine finally figured them out, and learned to share in the control they conferred. You can, too.

A few examples. When doctors make rounds, they know how many patients they must talk to. But patients and family members are rarely privy to this information. When a client sees a psychotherapist in his office, the client knows there are 50 minutes available, to be used however he or she wishes. When a patient or family member sees a doctor in the hospital, they have no idea how long the examination will take or how much time, if any, will be left for their questions. The doctor, as timekeeper, maintains total control over the interaction.

89

But if the patient or family member knows the unofficial rules—if they know enough to claim 10 minutes, say, of the doctor's undivided attention—they can use those rules to their advantage. They can contract with the doctor, literally as he comes through the door, for a piece of the action.

"I have several things to ask you," you might announce. "So it would help if you'd let me know how much time you need for your exam, and how much I can have for my questions." Once granted a stretch of time, no matter how short, you have license to take charge. During *your time*, you can direct all the verbal interaction.

For one thing, you can forestall doctor interruptions. Doctors often demonstrate that they have the upper hand by using subtle, often unconscious, forms of intimidation. According to linguist Joyce Neu of the University of Southern California, they interrupt patients twice as often as patients interrupt them. Verbal interruptions are frequently a form of social marker, a way to create a power imbalance. According to Neu, "Interrupting is a way for a physician to say he or she doesn't want to be questioned."

But if you've established your *own* ground rules, you've forestalled the interruptions before they start. If the doctor has previously agreed that you have 10 minutes to use in any way you choose, *you* can decide who talks and who doesn't. "Excuse me, doctor," you might interject, "but it's important for me to tell you how I feel. When I finish, I'll be interested to hear your reaction."

How else can you stake your claim to this time? Ask the doctor to sit down. Pediatricians are taught that they get better communication from their young patients if they are at eye level with them, even if that means getting down on stiff knees in the emergency room. Doctors treating adults know this principle, but ignore it. They usually stand halfway in the door, poised to escape as soon as possible. Katherine had used several methods to get the attention of Dr. Lloyd, following him down the hall, straining to establish eye contact. But not until she began insisting on contact on her own turf (in her father's room) and on her own time did she see real results.

Too close contact, on the other hand, can be equally harmful to a partnership. I have seen doctors lean or sit on beds, putting patients at a disadvantage with undue familiarity. I have seen them, through such carelessness, cause unnecessary physical pain around stitches and other sensitive areas. You needn't tolerate that. Your room is *your* space, not the doctor's. If you claim it as yours, you can set the tone.

Just think about it in terms of your home. If a physician or guest visited your home, they wouldn't stand in the door or sit on your bed. They would wait for you to offer them a chair. The key ingredient here is your attitude. Act as if this is your home, or you will forfeit it to others.

However, one note of caution. If your doctor has entered a time agreement, honor it. Don't extend a 10-minute consultation to 15 minutes. When he's met you halfway, don't ask for more. Don't chase him down the hall; don't approach him in elevators. Keep other family members off his back. If your family is large, arrange for a group consultation. Or select one individual as spokesperson, assigned to carry information back and forth.

If you need more time—and those making critical care decisions *do* need more than 10 minutes—ask for a longer session. If you need a half hour or more, offer to schedule time at the end of the working day or at the doctor's office. If you continually need more time than is customary in your hospital or community, offer to pay for a private consultation.

This last is crucial to selling the idea of the care partner program. One of the greatest fears of doctors is that, once patients and their families become interested and active, they will demand too much (unpaid) time. In my view, that fear is unjustified. A doctor's reluctance to spend extra time, especially at the outset of a patient/doctor relationship, is shortsighted. "Initially, encouraging a patient to ask questions *can* take more time," says Dr. Dean Edell, a San Francisco-based physician, who on his daily radio show encourages patients to become more active in their own care."But if a doctor thought about it for a second, he would realize that this early investment in education and training could prevent frantic calls in the middle of the night and extra time spent dealing with the same issues, over and over, visit after visit."

In short, a partnership works best when you and all the professionals you work with respect the problems and concerns of each other. If they respect your right and need to know, they profit from dealing with an informed patient who, by virtue of that knowledge, is more cooperative. If you respect the heavy demand on their time and demonstrate your desire to ease that demand, you profit from their greater willingness to "open up" during the time they spend with you.

PREPARING, LISTENING, LEARNING

Dr. Lloyd, glancing at his watch, noted that by now he should be finishing his third floor rounds. But waiting for him in the next room was that woman and her sister-in-law. Annoyed, he wondered what they wanted now. Were they going to slow him down?

But something about the way they approached him felt different. Katherine's questions, he had to agree, were legitimate. These were questions she couldn't look up on her own or take to the nurses. They were questions only he, the doctor, could answer.

Also, she'd apparently prepared for this meeting. She spoke from notes she seemed to have written down ahead of time.

Finally, they seemed determined to really get what he told them—and not forget it. Sarah was actually taking notes on his answers in their little green book.

No doubt about it, he mused, these two were a bundle of surprises. Maybe he was going to cover the third floor on time after all.

By being prepared for their doctor, by showing that they respected his time, but at the same time being determined to pursue their goal, Katherine and Sarah were beginning to gain his respect. Few patients and families think through these points. "My patients never come to me prepared," one family practitioner has told me. "If I needed to see an architect, I would study up before the appointment."

This doctor has a point. Before seeing our physician, we should have our facts in order—and where that isn't possible, have our questions ready. Doing our homework beforehand serves a dual purpose: It puts us on a more even footing with him, reducing the intimidation we may feel around a professional; and it helps us to help him save valuable time.

But our job doesn't stop with being armed with facts and questions. We need to listen carefully, so we can retain what we're told. When we meet our doctor prepared, we save some of his time. When we listen carefully and retain what he says, we save more of his time. So we need to formulate a plan—*before* he enters the room—for receiving the information he will give us.

Few people prepare such a plan. A constant complaint of physicians is that their patients don't hear them—that while they may ask good questions, they rarely hear the answers. I suspect the main reason for this is stress. Neither physicians nor patients fully realize how much stress is generated by medical interviews.

There are several ways to surmount this problem.

- *Invite a "Secretary:"* Here's a rough analogy, and a possible solution. Before my husband and I bought our word processor, we did some comparative shopping. Dealing with "computerese" was stressful for both of us. We had no prior knowledge to build on. We felt ignorant and out of our depth. After one sales pitch, I glanced at my husband. He looked like he'd been in the spin cycle of an automatic washer. I'm sure I looked the same. And neither of us could recall a word we'd heard.

  To deal with the problem, we devised a plan. One of us would interact with the salesperson and the equipment, while the other would jot down things to remember. It worked. We soon sorted out the information we needed to make our decision.

  The same strategy works in a medical interview. Invite a spouse or a friend to be your "secretary." Not having to take notes will free you to really listen to your doctor's answers. And your secretary's notes will provide you with detailed reminders, against which you can check your memory after the interview is over.

- *Use a Tape Recorder:* A tape recording serves the same purpose, perhaps even better. While using a recorder in a medical interview is considered unorthodox and usually requires prior permission, getting your information "right" and getting it "whole" is extremely important, particularly when the news is bad. Most people, on receiving word of a life-threatening condition, go into self-protective shock. Some do when hearing an unexpected prognosis. An audio recording allows them to listen to the information they need to understand at a later time, when their "anesthesia" has worn off and they can really hear it.

Another time when a tape recorder is useful is when all family members can't be present at a crucial interview or when a specialist is giving a medical evaluation. Your primary doctor, or other health specialists working with you but not at this session, may well benefit from such verbatim recordings.

- *Separate Answers From Questions:* When use of a tape recorder is not appropriate, and you must rely on hastily jotted notes, devise a system for separating questions from answers, so the latter won't get lost. One way is to write your prepared questions in ink and the doctor's answers in pencil. You may think of a better way. The exact method isn't important. What is important is to avoid the feeling you often have after leaving a party—that you were too busy plotting what you would say next to really hear what was being said to you.

- *Repeat Back What You Hear:* The simplest of all methods, requiring no equipment or special permissions, is to repeat back what you've heard at the end of the session. In just a few sentences you can summarize what you've learned, and the doctor can assess its accuracy. "So let me see if I understand what you've said," such a recital could start out. "My hypertension can be treated by the drug Inderal, which you plan to prescribe. But I should also lower the cholesterol and salt in my diet, cut out cigarettes, and limit my alcohol intake to 2 ounces a day."

95

UNDERSTANDING THE SYSTEM

"As best I can figure out, this hospital is organized something like this," Sarah said, *sketching hastily on a sheet of butcher paper. "On top is the Board of Directors. Then there're two administrative wings—the physicians' side and staff's side."*

As her red and blue felt pens flew across the page, her drawing began to resemble a family tree.

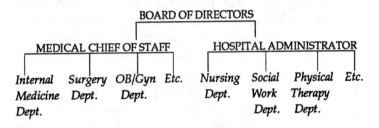

"Now," she said, *adding a last arrow down the side of the page, "let's figure out the people we should get to know."*

In a hospital, it seems a whole army of R.N.s, L.V.N.s, nursing aides, therapists, and technicians stream through our lives every 24 hours. And in most hospitals they come in three shifts—a different set of names, faces and temperaments every eight hours. Sometimes even those line-ups change from day to day.

Small wonder that we rarely know who is responsible for us and who can make a difference in our care. We're defeated from the start by a mysterious, multi-faceted "system." What's more, if we manage to learn how it works in one institution, we have to relearn it in the next, since each is slightly different from the last. So whether you're a patient or a family member, it behooves you to learn at the outset what *yours* looks like. Here's how.

- *Make Your Own Chart:* An organizational chart such as the one Sarah made will help you find your way around the hospital as a whole. But the service most crucial to a patient's daily welfare—and the one most difficult to understand—is the nursing service. With the aid of a chart, you can learn who is responsible for you, when and for how long. All you need to do is begin the chart and ask the first nurse who comes in to fill in the names. It might start out by looking something like this.

DIRECTOR OF NURSES—Dorothy Epstein

SUPERVISORS OF NURSING—
Constance McPhail, A.M.
Janine Jones, P.M.
Josephine Rutherford, Nights

HEAD NURSE MEDICAL/SURGICAL UNIT	STAFFING COORDINATOR	DR. OF EDUCATION
Charge — Barbara Barnes, A.M. *Nurses* — Harriette White, P.M — Joanne Anderson, Nights	*"Float Nurse" Coordinator*	*Clinical Nurse Specialists*
Staff Nurses _____ _____ _____ _____ _____	(Nurses assigned to units as needed)	(Specialized nurses, often used as counselors, health educators)
Licensed Vocational Nurses _____ _____ _____		
Nursing Aides _____ _____ _____		

97

- *Get to Know the Hierarchy:* While titles can vary from institution to institution, certain hierarchical patterns apply almost everywhere. In most nursing homes, and in hospitals like the one outlined above where "team nursing" is used, you will find a head nurse assigned to each floor or unit. While officially there only on the day shift (7 A.M. to 3 P.M.), that person is responsible for everything that happens on the unit and is usually called in when trouble arises, whatever the hour. During hours when the head nurse is not on the premises, direct supervisory responsibility rests with a charge nurse, the next person in the chain of command on that unit for that day. Different charge nurses are usually assigned to the afternoon and the evening shifts.

  With "total care nursing," a nurse is assigned daily to a group of patients. That nurse studies the charts, writes the care plans and has responsibility for the "total care" of the patients assigned to her that day. With "primary care nursing," the *same* nurse is assigned to the *same* set of patients each day for total nursing care until those patients are *discharged* from the unit.

  In all systems, nursing supervisors, clinical nurse specialists and "float nurses" operate throughout the hospital. Since they can be called for special assignment to any floor, it is helpful to identify them as well.

- *Speak to the Right Person:* One of the prime reasons for getting to know staffing systems is to learn who has the authority to make decisions in your hospital. Once you know that, you know the right people to talk to—the people who can make a difference. Even good assertive communication, when directed to the wrong person, rarely gets you what you want. Here are some guidelines for focusing on the people who count.

With "team nursing" you should start with the head nurse or charge nurse on your floor. Under this system, rarely should unusual treatment information or administrative decisions be sought through staff nurses or others further down the hierarchy. "Staff nurses are leary about talking about these things with families, and with just cause," a head nurse explained to me. "If they don't tell the families what they know, the families get upset. If they do, the doctor and other nurses get upset. It's a tough situation. If you want to know who to go to, it's your head nurse, charge nurse, the supervisor or the director of nurses. They would feel most comfortable sitting down talking with you."

On the other hand, with "primary nursing" or "total care nursing," you *should* start with the nurse assigned directly to your care. If for any reason you are not satisfied with the results, then you can go up the ladder to the next person in charge.

Another set of people you should get to know well—for very different reasons—are the nursing aides. Although some acute care facilities are moving away from hiring aides, many still do. And intermediate and long-term care facilities still rely heavily on their services. Within these health care centers, aides often give you the most "hands-on" care. They bathe you, feed you, change your sheets and empty your bedpan. In some institutions, they're the only staff directly assigned to you. Because you spend more time with them than anyone else, you have more chance to cultivate their friendship. Do so if you can. They can be, and often are, your staunchest allies.

AVOIDING OVERKILL

Once you've learned your way around the hospital and found how successful you can be with assertive techniques, you may be tempted to overplay your hand. You may discover that you enjoy the adversarial role and are using these tactics frequently, sometimes just for the excitement they bring.

To understand what's happening here, we need to make a distinction. When patients and families feel they are being bullied by professionals, they sometimes bully back. But the angry, hostile reaction discussed earlier in this book is usually the kind generated by a sense of *powerlessness*. The aggressive and belligerent behavior mentioned here is a direct *misuse of power*.

Avoid overkill. When overly assertive strategies are applied too many times in hospitals, especially against entrenched "experts" who will always have the edge on an "outsider," a fruitless, sometimes catastrophic, power struggle usually ensues, one which the "outsider" almost always loses.

To prevent this from happening to you, remind yourself of the responsibilities that accompany your newfound rights. Carry this rule around with you: *Do what you must do to get what you need in a hospital, but not in a way that unjustly attacks health professionals or prevents them from doing their job.* Monitor yourself for any patronizing tones in your voice, any appearance of stubbornness or irritation. Be quick to acknowledge your doctor's, nurse's, technician's areas of competence. And when possible, take time out for reflection. Carefully judge this interaction and answer these questions: Will this get me what I want in quality care? Or is it essentially a power struggle, one in which my real object is to overcome my opponent?

If the answer to the first question is "no," and to the second "yes," ask yourself a third question. Does this exchange *have* to be adversarial? Is there another way?

In a care partnership, there is. Think of your interactions with the other members in your triad as a dance. In a well-executed ballet, power isn't fought over, it's merged. Energies aren't dissipated in anger, they're blended.

But the subtleties of this exchange are rarely learned through another's words. They must be *felt* through your *own* actions. In a workshop I once conducted on leadership, I asked participants interested in learning co-leadership skills to choose a partner. Then I told them to do these things:

- Stand facing one another. Take a deep breath from the abdomen and relax. Feel yourself centered and grounded.

- Assign one partner to be the leader, and begin with any movement that person chooses to initiate.

- The other partner should follow closely, imitating the movement. The follower should pay close attention to the leader. Keeping eye contact and total body awareness, the follower should create a mirror image of what the leader is doing.

- Now, switch roles. The person who has been the follower should become the leader. Repeat the process, but in reverse.

- After a while, begin to change roles on your own, the leader becoming the follower and vice versa in natural alternations until you are moving smoothly together without conscious thought.

- You should find—and this is the point of this exercise—that in time you will shed your leader-follower identities. You will jointly sense the next movement to make. And together you will make it.

101

This may seem overly fanciful in the hospital context. And of course it is—if you're taking what I'm saying literally. Obviously you're not about to ask your doctor for the next dance. But note how similar to my workshop instructions are my guidelines for building a good care partnership.

The sequence of events is basically the same. Pay attention to the other person. Listen to what is being said. Watch his or her body language. Notice how he or she walks, talks, breathes. For a while, at least, try being as much like this partner as possible. Then, at the appropriate moment, take charge of what's happening between you. Initiate movement on your own, but not of an alien nature. Build on the groundwork already laid by your partner. But invite him or her to move one step further, to extend your joint energy one notch higher.

There's a saying that it's easier to ride a horse in the direction it's going. In aikido, you use the energy of your partner to propel yourself forward. In dance, you anticipate and complement the movement of your partner. And as you do, something happens. As you move with someone else, physically or emotionally, you build rapport. As rapport deepens, trust and understanding follow. When that occurs, all partners are set free to lead *and* follow. They become equal members of a true partnership.

Chapter 5

TRANSCENDING
THE SYSTEM

Katherine watched her aunt pick out the prisms, some tear shaped, some flat with cut glass patterns worked throughout. Looking at them, she thought of words from a poem she'd once heard.

> Love is to life,
> As after is to rain;
> I've seen it pass through
> Birth and death
> Make prism out of pain.
> —Victoria Forrester
> "So Penetrant a Light"
> A LATCH AGAINST THE WIND

Reaching high in the window frame, Aunt Dorothy began to hang the shimmering prisms, one by one, so that each would take advantage of any sunlight coming through John's new room on the medical unit. Room 203 was a small, utilitarian space, furnished in *standard "hospital modern." It had a green naugahyde chair in the far corner, a formica side table with imitation wood grain next to the bed. And that was about it.*

Struggling to get used to their four walls, the family, supplemented now by the arrival of John's sisters to help during the holidays, had done what they could to make prisms from their pain. A sunflower print on the wall. An oval rug with blue, green and gold fabrics braided through it. Light, airy curtains. A bird feeder already attracting sparrows at the window sill. And now these prisms, gathering up the morning sunlight and flinging it about the room in a thousand flecks of brilliant color.

What surprised Katherine was how easy it had been. How much light there'd been around them, once they'd looked for ways of catching and reflecting it. How much beauty had come through their broken edges—when they'd let it happen.

Individualized, integrated care, respectful of our past, present and future. It's what we all want. It's what Katherine's family wanted. They wanted to see John's emotional, social and spiritual needs assigned equal status with his physical ones.

Madison County Hospital was as good as any hospital, perhaps better than most. But if the hospital had been responsible for delivering this type of care, it simply wouldn't have happened.

Yet hospitals all over the country make an enormous effort to ensure that a certain level of care is accorded to all patients. Peer reviews and quality assurance checks serve to guarantee that each patient gets a designated level of quality care. Equality is the watchword. But as necessary as it is, equality can have a grim leveling effect. Standard care for everyone usually means individualized and special care for none.

DOING IT YOURSELF

They'd begun to realize the possibilities the day they tackled their father's room. Katherine and Sarah ransacked the family photo album, picking out shots of John as an active, vibrant man—golfing, mowing his lawn, feeding his dog, playing with his grandchildren.

They assembled the elements of a family tree, choosing pictures of his parents, of his children, of their children."Where do you think this one should go?" Katherine asked Sarah, holding up one of John with his only granddaughter."Why not put them all right above his head," Sarah said with sudden inspiration, "so people will have to get close to him to see them."

If John's family hadn't taken the time to establish his identity, his value as a human being, who would have? Who on the staff would have personalized his care? Realistically, who could have?

A major irony of today's hospital scene is that while doctors and nurses become more and more trained in the psycho-social and spiritual needs of patients, they have less and less time to act on what they've learned. Frustrated, many health professionals leave the profession. Those who remain simply give up on the possibility of a holistic environment in a hospital setting.

I know many fine holistic doctors who have found a way to deal with this dilemma. They no longer seek hospital privileges. If they can't be the kind of physician they want to be *in hospitals*, they limit their practices to patients who stay *out of them*. But while this may work well for these doctors, it clearly fails for their patients who fall acutely ill.

As long as people need hospitals, it is irresponsible of us to abandon the struggle to make hospitals more humane. In the past we haven't known how, but now care partnering offers a philosophy and a structure to help us at least begin.

"I realized there was little I could do to change the outcome of my husband's illness," said one care partner I knew whose husband had multiple sclerosis. "But something in me said there was a way I could change the hospital experience."

IT'S SO EASY

The most important care partner principle, and one I've never known to fail, is simply this: To *attract* outstanding care for those you love, the care partner must *give* outstanding care—to everyone who walks into the room. And what you'll find is, *it's so easy.*

Because of your sensitive involvement and practical help, hospital workers find that routine physical care takes less time. And because of the extra appreciation you accord them when you see what they do close up, they find themselves renewed and energized, able to perform their jobs with more pride and pleasure.

But how to begin? I can tell you about other patients, other care partners. And I do in the next section. But in the end, you must write your own healing story. Doctors and nurses may be the experts on physical care, but only you can fashion the care that starts where physical treatment leaves off. Your individualized approach will set the tone. You will determine the content of your program and its level of intensity, based on what has meaning for you. It's not *what* you do or *how much* you do that really matters, but whether what you do has significance to you as it develops. The secret of success lies in *your* creative energy, your deeply felt, ongoing process.

THE CREATIVE PROCESS

Let's look at a few stories. Probably our country's best known "creative patient" is Norman Cousins, former editor of the *Saturday Review*, and writer and lecturer on methods for staying well. While fighting a collagen disease in 1964, Cousins took charge of his own healing environment. Sixteen years later, following a serious heart attack, he applied the same formula. With his doctor's help, he built a program around the positive emotions of love, hope, faith, laughter, confidence and the will to live. He became his own care partner.

His treatment for collagen disease, now widely known and respected, included ten minutes of laughter every day. He watched old Marx Brothers' films and Allen Funt's "Candid Camera" television shows. He read humorous books by Max Eastman and E. B. White. And what he found was that ten minutes of belly laughter during the day almost always gave him two hours of painless sleep at night.

He also found that his laughter treatments produced a five-point drop in his sedimentation rate, confounding doctors' predictions that his disease—in their view irreversible—would produce total paralysis in five years. Five years later he was not only not paralyzed, he was cured.

Rosa Browning, a woman in her eighties, was not recovering from open heart surgery. Each day she was getting weaker, and those close to her were certain she was dying. One day while visiting Rosa, a friend asked, "Who makes you feel good to be around?" She suggested that Rosa visualize these people visiting her in her convalescent hospital room.

As Rosa began listing names, her spirits seemed to lift. Some of her old vitality returned. Just remembering the people who had always given her pleasure appeared to revive her will to live. A nurse noting the change took Rosa's friend aside and urged, "Whatever you're doing, keep it up. Not only can I see it in her face, her vital signs are responding, too."

In a few days Rosa and her friend had devised what they called "Rosa's Get-Well Project." A list of 31 names had soon come together—some close friends, some long-time acquaintances. But Rosa didn't limit herself to these. She listed everyone she felt might help, regardless of how close the relationship. Some were people she barely knew. But in one way or another they'd had some positive influence on her life.

A letter was sent to them letting them know that. In it, they were asked to make a three-month commitment to help Rosa "get well." Each was requested to sign up for one day a month. "On your day," the letter suggested, "you might call Rosa and ask her what she needs. Some days she might need shopping done. Some days she might need someone to talk to. She might ask you to read poetry to her. She might like a home cooked meal. Ask her what she had to eat yesterday, and what type of menu seems appetizing today."

A few days later, these 31 people, mostly strangers to one another, came together for a kickoff party. They met to ask questions, get answers, prepare plans, but mainly to dedicate themselves to an important project.

Within two weeks, Rosa was out of the hospital, and within three months she was recovering. The cardiac surgeon had performed the operation, but Rosa, with the intervention of her nurse and the help of her friends, had conducted her own healing.

In an article published in *Medical Economics*, Caroline Driver, whose husband Bob had leukemia, told how she decorated his hospital room to look as much as possible like home. She brought in carpeting from their living room, colored pillow cases from their home, photographs and posters, books, a stereo system. And since Caroline stayed with Bob around the clock, she installed an electric frying pan so she could do simple home cooking. Though her meals couldn't be too ambitious, they could be elegant. And they often were, right down to the chilled wine served in heirloom blue glasses.

When they wanted privacy, Caroline and Bob placed a "Don't Disturb" sign on the door. In short, they refused to be institutionalized. They remained the same Mr. and Mrs. Driver in the hospital as they had been at home.

On August 11, 1973, the *San Francisco Chronicle* reported another such story.

"For almost as long as she has been able to remember, Ruth Hoffman has liked parties.

"She liked to give them. She liked to attend them. And for years as part of a string ensemble, she used to play at them.

"Today, between noon and 8:00 p.m., Mrs. Hoffman, 57, will be hostess of what probably will be her last party.

"She is dying of cancer and she is having an open house in her room at Sequoia Hospital in Redwood City to bid her family and friends farewell."

In a later edition, the newspaper reported that the party had been a huge success—food, friends, laughter, memories and a radiant hostess.

These stories may not appeal to you. You may not like parties or your wife's cooking. You may not think the Marx Brothers are funny. You may not be an organizer and fighter. You may have limited resources, few if any loved ones and no privacy in your hospital room. But you do have your own style. And you can find some way, however modest, to express it. Some way to invoke *your* unique creative process.

109

CREATIVITY HEALS

The family gathered around John's bed. One of his two sisters was returning that morning to Atlanta, to her job and family responsibilities. And it was clear that this marked the beginning of many comings and goings. Family members relieving one another, weighing the imperatives of personal lives against the demands of a vigil that could last for weeks, months. Conducting some kind of ritual as people went seemed a way to give them a sense of closure, so they could grant themselves permission to leave.

They joined hands—tentatively at first, then more firmly as they felt the warmth of human contact—and their collective energy acted like an electric current coursing through the circle, melding them into a single force.

John's favorite scripture filled the room. Katherine closed her eyes, concentrating her love directly on her father. She visualized his body bathed in radiant light as he absorbed the intensity of these powerful words. "And now abideth faith, hope, and love, these three," their minister read in his clear, vibrant voice, "but the greatest of these is love."

The McGuire family employed this ritual every time there was a departure from the family team. The use of prayer, the reading of scripture, the communion as a family, each had a meaning important to them.

For other patients and families, different approaches will be more appropriate. The important thing is to invest what you do with personal conviction—because what we're talking about here is the power of mind and spirit over matter.

The mind affects the body. Creativity affects the body. When we focus our minds and direct our creative energies, we can have the same potent effect as does the sun when its rays are directed through a magnifying glass.

110

We generate energy naturally. Our choice is whether this energy is focused in constructive or in destructive ways. Worrying is one example of our creativity operating in the destructive mode. While all of us visualize, often we do it in negative ways. When we are diagnosed with heart disease, we are quick to choose negative images—the next heart attack, the Coronary Care Unit, the crash cart, sudden death. But when we consciously opt for positive imaging, we can focus on a healthy heart—on clear arteries, strong cardiac muscles, a happy and healthy life.

Several medical researchers are studying the effects of visualization on the body. Dr. Carl Simonton, a radiation oncologist, and Stephanie Matthews-Simonton, a psychotherapist, pioneered the early research in the area of visualization and cancer growth. Other practitioners soon followed. "Visualization is not wishful thinking, there is nothing magical about it," reports Dr. Dean Ornish, medical researcher at the University of California Medical School and author of *Stress, Diet and Your Heart*. "Neither is it daydreaming or fantasizing, both of which are unfocused and passive. Visualization is different from these—it is active and direct . . .Visualization gives you the power to direct internal processes somewhat. This can cause physiological changes to occur."

Images and associations selected by patients themselves are the most effective. One cardiac patient with whom I work—and who is in Dr. Ornish's current study—recently had to have surgery. With a seven-hour operation for prostatic cancer scheduled, he was told he could expect significant blood loss. His first response was to take some practical steps, lining up offers from donors with the same blood type, then donating one pint of his own blood. After that, he worked on his mind.

For weeks before the operation, using a visualization method, he pictured the incision. Then he imaged the blood moving away from it, actually drying up like a river in a very hot desert. And when the day of the operation came, not only did he come through the surgery and his recovery period ahead of schedule, he required no blood transfusions at all. His surgeons merely returned his own pint of blood as a protection and a courtesy.

Dr. Bernie Siegel, a cancer surgeon in New Haven, Connecticut, and author of *Love, Medicine and Miracles*, tells how the creativity of a husband positively affected his sick wife. The wife was suffering intensely from chemotherapy. Her nausea was so bad that her husband always had a brown paper bag ready after treatments so she could vomit into it. But one day he surprised her with something she loved. When she reached for her vomit bag, she found inside a dozen long-stemmed red roses.

The roses did their job. While she underwent many more chemotherapy treatments, she never again associated them with nausea—and they never again made her ill.

But red roses in paper bags don't work for every patient. An effective care partner program must be specific to the needs, wishes and preferences of the individual patient involved. Which only confirms a contention made earlier in this chapter—that healing doesn't come from the action taken, but from the activation of the patient's unique creative process. Or the healing can even come from the effect of someone else's creativity acting on the patient.

Psychologist Rollo May, in *My Quest for Beauty*, confirms this. Writing about his own clinical depression, he describes how he used the beauty of a field of poppies to heal himself. "A new quality of life which had begun with (drawing and listening to) the poppies had spread out to an awareness of

112

the colorful and adventurous aspect of life—the aspect of beauty—which had been there all the time but which I had never noticed. I seemed released from my old compulsions. I felt empowered, freed for all kinds of activities."

Science provides support for this theory. Endocrinologists believe that creativity produces brain impulses that stimulate the pituitary gland, and in turn the whole endocrine system. "Creativity for Pablo Casals was the source of his own cortisone," Norman Cousins wrote in his book *Anatomy of an Illness*. Citing the amazing longevity of the great cellist, Cousins theorized, "It is doubtful whether any anti-inflammatory medication he would have taken would have been as powerful or as safe as the substances produced by the interaction of his mind and body."

Could it be that this is the secret of healing? Creating an image, a ritual, a loving environment, a personalized care plan for ourselves or for someone we love? If so, one way to start is to get back in touch with our senses.

COMING TO OUR SENSES

In the evening they often sat around John's bedside, softly singing popular ballads from the past, harmonizing on the familiar parts, humming through the ones they couldn't recall. Often the nurses and the aides would join them, supplying a missing word or a lost phrase.

Aunt Dorothy remembered the old songs—"Steamboat Round the Bend," "Marie," "Moonglow"—that had touched John's childhood and adolescence. Each person in the circle knew a different era, knew songs from different times in John's life, evoking different memories and different tears.

Katherine remembered the music of the 1940s—when she was a

113

young child and John a young father. He'd taught her the alphabet with music, he and Perry Como. "'A'—You're Adorable," he and Perry sang as they covered the ABC's.

Now, as he lay in a coma, she called upon those simple ballads, hoping something might touch a nerve somewhere."Remember this one, Daddy? About fairytales that come true? It can happen for you . . . I know it can."

A creative impulse translated into action. Care tailored to the sensibilities and needs of John McGuire and nobody else. And so simple. I'm often asked for concrete ways to introduce creative care partnering to a hospital setting—natural, organic forms of care that can apply to everyone, but be custom-tailored to each one. And the approach I always cite first is the most basic: Nourish the senses.

We usually thrive when these stimuli are present, and almost always languish when they're not. So why not use them to transform your hospital or nursing home? I invite you to let your imagination roam. For now, at least, don't worry about institutional approval. Just concentrate on your environment, making it a place of beauty, playfulness and whimsy, of sights, sounds, smells, tastes and touching.

Sights

John lay, day after day, his face turned to one side, eye patches in place to protect his corneas, seemingly deaf, mute and blind. But during quiet moments when they were alone, his remaining sister would describe the prisms to him—the rainbow glow they cast on the room, the delicate patterns they etched across the walls, their sudden shimmering movement when a breath of air rustled among them.

114

What is beautiful to you? A work of art, a spray of flowers, sunlight coming through a window, an old fishing hat, a favorite teddy bear or blanket? At Planetree, care partners have brought in banners, posters, family photographs, video movies, stained glass. Shirley MacLaine, in the film *Terms of Endearment*, hung an original Renoir where her daughter, dying of cancer, could see it from her bed. Katherine introduced growing plants, a bird feeder, prisms, carefully selected television programs. Though John couldn't see the programs, there was a chance he could hear them. And the images they suggested—the beauty of Joe Montana throwing a long forward pass, or Jack Nicklaus completing a 300-yard-drive—could be therapeutic.

Decorating rooms for patients too ill to open their eyes needn't be futile. The blind can experience beauty; they feel the effect beauty has on those around them. This is especially true of the beauty of color. Some researchers believe that color has such healing qualities that the sick will actually crave to be near certain tones and hues. The body may need color in the same way that it needs nourishing foods.

Sunlight, of course, contains all the colors. If you're lucky enough to have windows in your hospital room, and particularly if you have a southern exposure, this is a sensory pleasure easily available to you. If not, you can introduce your own colors. One care partner helped her loved one resist standard "hospital issue" and remain in colorful gowns of her own choosing. Slits down the backs and satin ribbons sewn around the necks transformed blue, yellow and pink flannel gowns, brought in from the outside, into functional hospital wear. I've heard of another patient who had hospital gowns made from his favorite plaid hunting shirts.

Whenever I think of a close friend who was once very ill, I always see her lying under her grandmother's heirloom quilt, a sea of multi-colored squares intersected by snowy white and bordered by sunshine yellow.

Sounds

One of John's friends had organized a group of men to pay regular visits to the hospital. Hearty outdoor men, all of them avid golfers, they were instructed to dress in their golfing clothes and to talk about John's favorite sport to him. Some even brought golf books and magazines to read aloud.

"Move your head the least little bit while you are stroking your putt," read Sam Harper, a tall grey-haired man dressed in plaid pants and Izod shirt, "and you lose all chance of accuracy." Their voices, radiating sunshine and fresh air, filled the room with an almost tangible male energy and with the kind of talk John liked best. If John didn't hear those voices, surely he felt them.

Health professionals usually tell you that hearing is the most receptive sense during severe illness and, in terminal situations, the last sense to go. In the case of someone like John, it may offer the only opportunity to reach the patient. Sounds can actually affect the brain, stimulating glands and tissue.

Music is even more powerful. Some post-stroke patients who can't speak can sometimes sing. Brain-damaged patients, unresponsive to other stimuli, can sometimes respond to music.

For most of us, sounds can be healing. As children, we were quieted and calmed by lullabies. As adults, we're renewed and uplifted by great music. Other cultures have known this for centuries. Native Americans have relied on chants. Tibetan monks have used tones for healing and for reaching deeper levels of consciousness. Yogis teach us that the sound "Om" does not *mean* peace, it *creates* peace through its sound vibrations. Sufis believe the sounds of their sacred chants and dances are as important as the meanings attached to those sounds. They believe there is an eternal, divine aspect to every sound, and that this is the quality which opens the heart to receive love and healing.

Of course, we all respond to sound differently. Listen to the hospital sounds around you—buzzers, beepers, voices calling out to other voices in the hallway. Some will be reassuring and soothing, others jarring, depending on your personal sensitivities. Discover which ones have positive and which have negative effects on you. Then try your hand at some modest sound engineering. You may want poetry or literature read to you. Or you may choose music or relaxation tapes. If I were the patient, I would choose meditation music. My children would opt for rock. When recorders are provided with ear phones, as at Planetree, patients can have their choice.

Many patients prefer silence. All Sufi chants and dances end with extended moments of silence. Quiet is essential for physical and spiritual healing. The yogis agree. They believe vital energy is lost through unnecessary speech. For this reason, visitors to a sick room should avoid small talk unless the patient initiates it. When the patient indicates, through words or body language, that he or she is fatigued or no longer interested, silence should be restored immediately. This is particularly important when more than one visitor is in the room. Conversation among visitors which does not include the patient should be avoided unless strongly encouraged by the patient.

Especially when a patient is in a coma or under anesthesia, the family should remind the staff to observe silence or speak directly to the patient in positive and reassuring ways. This request is best written up by the patient and hospital partners in the care partner agreement or submitted by the patient to the operating room staff in writing before surgery takes place.

Just remember, words and sounds are not necessary for deep communication to take place. Physical presence alone is a powerful communicator, sometimes made even more effective when accompanied by meditation, silent prayer or healing thoughts.

Smells

It was Sarah who thought of the shaving lotion. When they first took on the job of shaving John, they followed standard hospital procedure. Once over with an electric shaver. If the skin was dry, some medicinal lubricant. One day Sarah suddenly stopped, Norelco in hand, and said, as if reasoning to herself, "You know, the thing that always comes to mind when I think of John is the wonderful scent of his shaving lotion. Just because he's in the hospital, he doesn't have to smell like one. Why can't he smell like himself?"

If your patient can't tell you what aromas to introduce to the hospital room, take a cue from his or her past preferences—a favorite shaving lotion or perfume are just two possibilities. Or ask yourself what *you* like to smell. Fresh flowers? Baked bread? Scented candles? But remember that, as with sound, everyone's response to scent is different. What may please you, the care partner, may be offensive to the patient. Incense, for example, may give one person contentment and another sinusitis. Also, be aware that illness may change a person's experience of smell. What was once pleasurable may now be just the opposite.

In general, whether you provide new aromas in gentle moderation or stick to past preferences, trust your instincts. They're usually pretty good indicators.

Tastes

"Imagine yourself at home eating your favorite meal— chicken and dressing, tossed salad, stuffed potatoes and caramel cake." John had been in a coma for eight days now. It had been a long time since he'd tasted any food at all. But Katherine thought he might, at least, enjoy the memory. "And on Christmas Day, you liked Mother's eggnog with freshly grated nutmeg."

Sometimes we have to rely on our imagination—and often a wry sense of humor—to compensate for the loss of our favorite taste treats. But if the pleasures of eating and drinking are still available to you, prepare a menu. While some things on it may be unrealistic, others may not be. Most hospitals offer a choice of menus. And if there's a care partner arrangement, plates and utensils can be brought from home to make institutional fare look like home cooking.

Sometimes an extra tray can be ordered, so family members and patient can eat together. Perhaps special food can be brought in from the outside. Or, through the use of a grounded electric skillet, arrangements might be made for simple home cooking. At Planetree, care partners sometimes cook for their patients in the unit kitchen, where it's not unusual to come upon a group of them swapping recipes for "protein smoothies" or "eggplant parmesan."

What makes your mouth water? What was the special "sick food" your mother brought you as a child? Chicken soup? Popsicles? I remember a cancer patient who wanted to be rolled to the family waiting room to enjoy rice pudding. And even when she could no longer eat, she craved the freshly brewed coffee which her husband perked and fed her with a spoon. Those around her felt she sometimes got more relief from her husband's coffee than from her doctor's morphine.

Touching

> December 20—McGUIRE FAMILY LOG
>
> 6:30 P.M.—*Dad's breathing very loud and labored. Heavy perspiration. Nurse had to change bedclothes.*
>
> 7:10 P.M.—*Patted him for 15 minutes. Breathing became regular, perspiration normal.*

Nurses have always known the value of therapeutic touch. And families I work with often utilize its healing potential. Patting, hand holding and personal grooming are just a few of the simple, natural ways it can occur. Smooth bed linens and fluffed-up pillows, both invoking the positive power of touch, can bring enormous relief to a bedridden patient.

After a little training, most care partners are able to perform nursing tasks that both assist the staff and bring therapeutic benefits of touch to the patient. By learning passive range of motion exercises, they can help limber joints and muscles. Through regular turning of very weak patients to different positions, they can ward off bed sores and pneumonia. As their patients grow stronger, they can work with ambulation to build body endurance and avoid muscle atrophy.

Although massage must be done with care, so as not to loosen blood clots or do harm to recovering organs, limbs or

120

joints, certain massage techniques can be undertaken simply and effectively by care partners (with approval of doctor, nurse or physical therapist). Long, even strokes can be accompanied by soothing verbal images ("feel the ocean waves swell and release"). Outward movements from torso to fingers or from torso to toes can suggest that pain is leaving the body through its extremities. Body lotions can be used in conjunction with the physical movement.

The most effective way to calm anxious patients of all ages is to hold them. I once saw a very astute nurse approach a cancer patient's husband. "Your wife needs to be held," she told him. "It would help her more than anything. And none of us on staff can do it."

This nurse understood that husbands and wives, close relatives or friends can offer means of healing that, if practiced by the hospital care team, might be viewed as unprofessional.

What feels good to you? Can you ask for it? Can you accept it when others offer it to you? Touch is our natural way to share our love and our sexuality. For a person whose body and body-image have changed, it is the best way I know to show that your feelings for that person have not changed.

THREE RECOMMENDATIONS

By suggesting that you use the five senses as the basis for a hospital care partner program, I've invited you to let your imagination range freely, to be outrageous—at least at the outset. Now let me add some practical guidelines.

- *Allow the patient final say over what is done.* When the two of you disagree, give in gracefully. If the patient

121

is unable to express an opinion, think of yourself as acting on his or her behalf, steering the program along lines that you know he or she would approve.

What this means is that you should focus close attention on the patient at all times, watching to see how each intervention is greeted. Look out for fatigue. With seriously ill or very weak patients, you can ask for a nonverbal sign—a blink, a nod, a squeeze of the hand. Always watch for unsolicited reactions—any sudden changes on the electrical monitor or in temperature or blood pressure. Finally, use your silent modes of communication (meditation, prayer, whatever) as ways to receive responses. The important thing is to stay closely attuned.

- *Keep a check on the family dynamics.* Are different factions within the family fighting for power and control? There are hospital rules especially designed to protect patients from warring family members. And often they are sorely needed.

  Do you find yourself angry much of the time with another family member, the patient, the staff? This is a common reaction to crisis and stress. Ask the medical social worker, your minister or a counselor for help. Getting outside assistance is sometimes the most constructive gift you can give to everyone. But avoid at all costs dumping your emotional garbage in the sick room, where it may undermine the good work you've been doing. If you don't, you will soon find your visiting time (and other people's as well) restricted by staff.

- *Test your ideas for feasibility.* I encourage a "responsible/idealistic" approach. First consider what you want in its ideal form. The sky should be the limit. Then consider the technical and logistical problems this could pose. Safety problems, for instance. All electric appliances and flammable materials should be checked out with the head nurse and/or hospital engineer. Space restrictions and housekeeping requirements should be taken into account. And other patients quartered nearby must be considered, especially regarding sound. The list could go on.

None of this is to suggest undue compromise. But it does suggest caution. Consider the possibility that you may need a private room. Or you might try arranging for a cooperative roommate who is open to trying the same program.

BREAKING THE RULES *WITH* STAFF SUPPORT

What I'm suggesting may look like encouragement to break some hospital rules. Actually I'm suggesting more than that—I'm suggesting that you transcend the rules, mobilizing staff to support you in breaking rules that make no sense.

But to bring about change in long-standing rules—so that everyone is a winner and nobody a loser—you must get inside the heads of those who feel, initially at least, that they have something to lose. We've already touched on this theme: how fear of the unknown can afflict staff as much as it can patients and families; how breakdowns in communication and destructive patterns of behavior can persist on both sides. And in all these instances, we've found that a major remedy lies in understanding problems from the other person's point of view.

123

If you are a patient or a family member, look at things from the staff's perspective. If you are the doctor, look at them from the nurse's viewpoint; if a nurse, from the administrator's.

Consider the excessive workload in hospitals. Rules help to set boundaries around this workload, fend off unanticipated difficulties, and foster a sense of order and control. While rules are normally thought of as patient protection, they serve to protect staff as well. So when they're violated, it's not surprising that staff becomes uneasy.

"When you have any situation you're not used to dealing with—when you have someone acting differently—it unnerves the staff," said a social worker in a hospital where I once consulted. Given this fact, consider what staff must have thought of Katherine and Sarah, at least in the beginning. Posters? Prisms? Family Log Books? These people are out of line!

A threatened change in the status quo is especially frightening to those who enjoy prerogatives of rank and authority long associated with the present system. That's why, in order to effect change, you must convince the person you approach that your way of doing things will not threaten anyone's position within the established order; and that far from creating additional work and problems, it can actually reduce them. Better yet, try to persuade that person that it is possible to carry out your ideas within the framework of the existing system.

GETTING WHAT YOU WANT

Back at the beginning, Sarah had developed a special relationship with two of the nurses on staff. And before long, whether they were assigned to John McGuire or not, they were coming by every night to check up on Sarah and Katherine. The four struck up a friendship. But something else happened as well. In the most informal and natural way, the two nurses came to be John's primary nursing team.

"Sometimes families treat us like maids at the Holiday Inn," one of them remarked one day as she helped Sarah exercise John's arms and legs. *"But you all make us feel different. You make us feel sort of special."*

Getting what you want can be far less formidable than you at first imagine. In the beginning, building relationships with a whole army of hospital staff was extremely tiring and distracting for Katherine and Sarah. The absence of primary nursing at Madison County Hospital worked against the introduction of care partnering, even in the simplest forms. The fact that no one nurse felt primary responsibility for John McGuire's care, that the system was based on constantly rotating teams of strangers, was an enormous handicap.

To change that arrangement would have been difficult enough for someone working *inside* the system. For this family, coming in as outsiders, it seemed impossible. But in less than a week, the McGuire family had what many directors of nurses, even after years of struggling with charts and nursing meetings, never achieve—a system of consistent primary nursing care.

And the way it was brought about was so simple. *The family was grateful to these nurses for what they were doing, and Sarah and Katherine let them know it.* In response, these women became the family's advocates, translators, guides. Most significant for this discussion, the McGuire family got the advantages of primary nursing care for John without disturbing hospital routine, without threatening anyone's turf, without making waves that might have jeopardized their position in the hospital or their loved one's care.

YOU CAN HAVE IT BOTH WAYS

Last day at Madison County Hospital. Moving at 10 A.M. to Beaumont Valley Nursing Home. Katherine made her rounds of CCU, 1-West, Social Services, Physical Therapy, Respiratory Therapy, the Lab, the Financial Offices. "Well, things can get back to normal now," she told everyone. "We just want you to know how much we've appreciated everything you've done. You've made our time here special."

A nurse, pushing a cart of linens, appeared at the end of the hall. As she came closer, her thick red hair and level blue eyes looked familiar.

"We're gonna miss you," the nurse said as she came abreast of Katherine. "You know, you ended up helping us as much as you helped your father. I didn't think it'd work, but it did."

Suddenly she came from behind her cart. Walking directly up to Katherine, she threw strong, freckled arms around her neck. "I won't forget you. I may never see you again, but I won't forget you."

You may feel that you can't have it both ways—your program *and* a good relationship with staff. But, in fact, you can. When conditions are right, when a dual appeal is made to people's capacity for idealism and their sense of self-interest, attitudes can and do change. Staff-based treatment plans and family-based healing plans can coexist.

WHEN THE STAFF SAYS "NO"

If you encounter hurdles at first, simply work for compromise. Here's an instance where a family was at first told "no." At Marin General Hospital in Greenbrae, California, the parents of a child in the Intensive Care Unit wanted to decorate his room. The staff felt space was too limited to accommodate the necessary medical equipment and all the toys, books and photos the family wanted in. So the family proposed a compromise.

At certain prearranged times, family members would create an environment for their patient. The doors would open and they would walk in with colorful, helium-filled balloons and various love objects from the child's room at home. With the doctor's permission, a feast would be laid out, consisting of hamburgers from McDonald's. But as with Cinderella when the clock struck midnight, at the end of the ten-minute visiting time the hospital room would return to "normal."

The idea worked better than anyone had anticipated. Without interfering with hospital routine, the family had achieved an atmosphere of personalized love for the child. What they ultimately achieved was a sense of delight and anticipation for everyone involved, including staff. Through determination and sensitive negotiation, they had demonstrated that staff as well as patient and family could have the conditions they needed for the dual tasks at hand—treatment *and* healing.

HELPING THE STAFF SAY "YES"

Here are some guidelines that can help you transcend your hospital system:

- *Know what you want to do.* That may sound obvious, but many people really aren't sure. Develop a rationale, one you believe in, one you can commit to. This may require changes in the existing system, but if you are clear in your mind that it is absolutely beneficial to your patient, and if you've worked out the details of carrying it out with minimal disruption to the status quo, then go after what you want with firmness and determination.

- *If you are not used to asking for what you want, practice ahead of time.* Rehearse with others or in front of a mirror. Then, if assertiveness remains too difficult to attempt on your own, find yourself an advocate within the system—a nurse, the doctor, the social worker— someone who can speak for you and who will back you up in what you want to do. In fact, this person could well serve on your care partner team.

- *Get approval from the top.* When you've picked the professional for your care partner triad, he or she should be able to work your ideas through the system. If that doesn't happen, try this approach: First, seek approval for your program from the doctor in attendance. Then try to get this approval written into the patient's chart. It's also important to talk with the head nurse (A.M. shift) or the charge nurses (P.M. and evening shifts). With other nursing systems, ask the nurse assigned to you whom to approach to seek the authority you need. Often certain nurses can give permission without doctor's orders. But even when approval is not necessary, the courtesy of communication goes a long way towards winning support and preventing future problems.

  In general, doctors will approve psycho-social-spiritual plans (even if they do not value their importance) if you can convince them that the nurses won't be hassled. Doctors have to look after their own skins, too. And unhappy nurses don't make their lives any easier.

- *Establish your credibility.* Don't be viewed as a rebel, a generalized rule breaker. You are only interested in exceptions that could be beneficial to your patient. If studies show heart patients need quiet to heal cardiac tissue, don't ask for long visits in the CCU. On the other hand, if your husband is dying and no other patients are being disturbed, then your request for longer visits is a justifiable request that should be honored.

- *Build an atmosphere of mutual trust.* Only when the parties involved trust one another can change take place. Demonstrate that you possess the ability to handle what you propose or, when you have doubts, the good judgment to check it out with staff. Effective care partners are those who have confidence in what they *do* know, but aren't afraid to acknowledge what they *don't* know. In those cases where extended visiting hours are granted, pledge to the nurses—and to yourself—not to impede the physical care program in any way.

- *Be flexible.* Show your willingness to accept adjustments in your plan. Call it, and think of it, as a demonstration project. Be prepared to fine tune it as needed. And be willing, if it isn't working, to abandon it altogether.

- *Find the courage to say how important this program is to you.* In 1971, hospital rules forbade me to wear my glasses into the operating room for a C-section.

> *"But I need my glasses to see," I argued. "I know I can cooperate better with full vision."*
> *Silence from the hospital staff.*
> *"I'll sign any paper you give me absolving everyone of liability for injury, loss, infection, whatever."*
> *Again, silence.*
> *"I don't understand your logic. The doctor's glasses will be directly over the incision. Won't they pose more threat of infection than mine?"*
> *I was getting nowhere.*
> *Finally, I said, "It's very important for me to see my baby. I've had to forego a labor and a natural birth. Please know how much I need to see my baby at the moment of birth."*
> *I got to wear my glasses throughout the operation.*

When you expose your real feelings, your love and concern, and when you appeal to these same emotions in your listener, you can have a far greater impact, and at a deeper level, than that achieved by rational arguments alone. Moreover, the response you evoke can be more spontaneous, heartfelt and deeply gratifying for all parties concerned.

Through the open demonstration of your love and concern, you will have found the way to let beauty come through the broken edges of your pain. And the rainbow colors it casts will light up your life and the lives of everyone around. You will have found the way to transcend the hospital system.

Chapter 6

GIVING without GIVING OUT
or GIVING UP

PART I: RENEWING OURSELVES AND EACH OTHER

Well before it appeared, Katherine heard its thick rubber wheels rolling swiftly down the hallway. In her mind's eye, she saw its curved metal fittings streaking along under the fluorescent lights, its massive shape dodging people and obstacles, maneuvering around corners, moving inexorably toward her father's room.

Then it suddenly appeared in the doorway—the ambulance guerney, propelled by two strong young men in starched white uniforms. Quickly, silently, they surrounded her father's bed and prepared to lift him out of it.

Katherine hurried to his side and told him what was happening, how he would be rolled out the front door of Madison County Hospital and driven down Lexington Drive to Beaumount Nursing Home.

Her strong, steady voice belied her sinking spirits. In a few minutes, she'd be starting all over again in a new place. A whole set of strange nurses to be met and won over, new aides to be befriended, the physical therapist to be contacted, the administrator and social worker to be persuaded to give her a chance.

And all the time this numbing fatigue. She longed to drive home and sleep. But she felt she had to go on. She had to muster the strength to face the new staff.

"It's more blessed to give than to receive" we were taught by our elders, and some of us learned the lesson well. Too well. Those who are natural givers tend to give and give and give until we "give out" or "give up."

The givers of the world extend across all boundaries. Particularly numerous in hospital and nursing home settings (and on care partner teams), they're found in great numbers among health professionals and, when families are in medical crisis, among certain family members. Moreover, the perpetual givers staunchly believe that their opposites, the receivers, are as eager to receive as they are compelled to give.

But this is rarely true. Any locked-in behavior pattern, confined to a single way of responding, will eventually lead to deep discontent—in this case, for both givers and receivers. As for the care partner relationship itself, unilateral giving and receiving are deeply antithetical to it. Care partnering thrives only when the giving and receiving are reciprocal.

GIVING AND RECEIVING:
THE EITHER/OR SYNDROME

In a workshop I conducted a few years ago, I asked the participants to list situations in their lives where they had given when they didn't want to give or received when receiving went against the grain. Their responses were instantaneous.

"Giving to the United Fund at work."

"Receiving an enema."

"Taking the kids to Toy World."

"Listening to a boring lecture."

"Attending your own surprise party."

When I asked the workshop members to describe how they felt at these moments, they were fascinated to find, on recalling their emotions, that above all they felt powerless. At some level they felt out of control, because they were being forced to give or receive against their will.

Then I asked the workshop to recall some *positive* experiences with giving and receiving. Again they were in for a surprise. They found they'd usually approached giving and receiving with an "either/or" attitude. The process went something like this. Each individual had his/her own "comfort zone" on a spectrum running from intense activity to extreme passivity, from full independence to almost total dependence, from a need to control to a need to acquiesce. To put it another way, each had a favored spot on the leader-follower continuum from which they rarely, if ever, departed.

COMFORT ZONES: BAD FOR YOUR HEALTH?

Comfort zones are comfortable. That's why we cling to certain behaviors so persistently, even when they may be bad for our health. For instance, recall if you can an emergency, such as a parent's sudden illness, which required that something be done immediately. Remember how family members fell into place on the leader-follower spectrum. Perhaps your older brother, a "take charge" personality from his earliest childhood, set up a command post by his telephone—calling an ambulance to rush your mother to the hospital, notifying other family members, alerting neighbors to feed the cat and water the plants.

Perhaps as the nurse or doctor in the family, you immediately took up your usual caregiving chores, whether or not they were wanted or even needed. Your younger brother, on the other hand, became the follower, willing to help but unwilling to act until he'd been told exactly what to do.

Finally, your sister played her traditional role of resident hypochondriac. She suddenly became ill, joining the patient in leaning on your brother and you for nurturance and protection.

My workshop people, reflecting on their positions along this continuum, came to realize how much these "positionings" had affected all aspects of their lives. Depending on which position had been habitually occupied, people had become some variation on one of the two personality types—the "giver" or the "receiver." But few, if any, had learned to be both. If one mode of behavior had been dominant, the opposite had never developed. But—and this was the crux of our discovery—its exclusion, while useful in the short run, had ultimately, over time, produced frustration, dissatisfaction and a depletion of energy for everyone involved.

BECOMING "STUCK"

"Always being one or the other (leader or follower, teacher or student, giver or taker) can deplete your energy

134

and limit your horizons," declared Beyhan Lowman, cancer patient and subject of *A Spirit Soars, Beyhan's Journey*. "If we can see ourselves in a dual role—offering and receiving—I think we can turn our living with one another into a continuously nurturing process."

Unfortunately, few of us ever achieve that balance. And the reason seems to be in our lack of wholeness, our tendency to become "stuck" in one set of behaviors. At one end of the spectrum are the "givers," constantly compelled to help someone, almost *anyone*. Whether their help is needed or wanted is not important. These are the martyrs of the world, giving bountifully but rarely receiving gracefully.

Granted, their gifts many times do help others. But constant giving is almost always a mixed blessing, even to them. The upside is that their giving gives them something in return. It gives them the sense of being useful. And whether they realize it or not, it gives them control over others. The downside is that they wear themselves out. In the end, they leave the scene exhausted, often bitter, rarely gratified.

Comfortably ensconced at the other end are the "takers," apparently content to be taken care of, but rarely prepared to give care to others. They are the child adults—selfish, self-centered, always dependent, always wanting more. Like the "givers," they can manipulate others, shape events, get what they need over the short term. But over the long term they, too, are unhappy with the results.

Constant receiving, unrelieved by the experience of giving, almost always produces in the recipients low self-esteem and an underlying resentment against the very people they must depend on for their gifts. Open hostility or deep depression is often the result—anger at being perpetually relegated to the ranks of the sick and the helpless.

Most of us at the workshop just described—mainly

parents, teachers and civic leaders—tended to be "givers."
When I did the same exercise with health workers, the scales
tipped even more in that direction. The only time we felt
comfortable receiving was when we were ill. We could think
of very few other times when we were able to ask for help,
even when we needed help desperately.

Consider this exchange between Edith and Mildred, the
friend and the wife of a patient hospitalized for cancer
treatments.

> EDITH: How are you doing?
> MILDRED: Just fine.
> EDITH: Do you need anything?
> MILDRED: Can't think of a thing, thank you.
> EDITH: Are you sure?
> MILDRED: No, everything's fine.
> EDITH: Let me know if I can do anything.
> MILDRED: Thanks, I will.

A typical scene in any hospital corridor. But those who
respond in this way—and I count myself among them—are
liars. We lie because we're uncomfortable asking for what we
need. Giving without receiving, we become hopelessly out of
balance, and in the process undo all our "good works." Having adopted giving as our exclusive preserve, we have set the
stage for "giving out"—and, ultimately, for "giving up."

HOW HOSPITALS MAKE MATTERS WORSE

*Riding along in the ambulance, Katherine wondered how she
could take the load off herself. How she could call on the basic
goodwill of other people to share some of her burden. It struck her that*

one way might be to take friends at their word. If they really wanted to "do something," let them. More to the point, tell them how.

She recalled her first days at Madison County Hospital. How much love and energy had flowed out—and then gone to waste. Visitors had streamed through her father's room. Within three days, she'd seen more hometown people than in the entire 17 years since she'd left Tennessee. On the third morning, after a great resurgence of appetite, she'd asked for a chicken salad sandwich and a tall glass of orange juice. Word promptly got around town that those were her favorite foods; and with classic southern hospitality, friends and relatives had poured in bearing large plastic containers of chicken salad and styrofoam buckets of fresh orange juice chilled with crushed ice.

If only there'd been a way of receiving all that goodwill in another form. And some way of returning it. But this was the way it was always done in this small rural town. Bringing food was a tradition.

So chicken salad kept coming in—and just as surely, when the family had eaten all it could, chicken salad kept going home to the back of their refrigerator.

The traditional hospital setting tends to discourage reciprocal giving and receiving. Indeed, people are *encouraged* to adopt polarized roles, even those who, outside the hospital, are well-balanced individuals. Doctors, nurses, technicians, therapists are paid to be givers—first, last and always. While they're on duty, the comforts of receiving are considered off bounds. Family members with seriously ill loved ones are expected, at a less intense level, to follow suit. On the other hand, patients are confined to receiving. Until they fully recover, they must remain, regardless of their personal inclinations, dependent recipients.

The care partner program corrects this imbalance. It offers

ways for members of each segment of the care team to take care of themselves, to extend care beyond themselves, and to receive care from other segments.

In *A Spirit Soars*, Dr. Richard Evans, a radiation oncologist, tells how this happened to him while working with the patient Beyhan Lowman.

"It has been two years since I met Beyhan and looking back some things look clearer now than they did at the time they were happening. Beyhan was seen for consultation and ultimately for a course of radiation therapy, yet I never really felt like I was her doctor. I was often her student and always her friend and sometimes I just felt like a fellow traveller groping my way down some strange, new path. We talked about options, and she made her choices. It was something we did together, but, I never really felt like her doctor. Sometimes I wonder if she ever felt like my patient . . .

Ultimately, Beyhan died with her cancer. Now here I sit trying to explain something that I don't really understand myself. My belief system has been rearranged and I can't get it back together just the way it was. I really don't want to. I find comfort in believing that we do have choices, that caring does make a difference, that love exists inside all of us. It is a lesson in life that Beyhan helped me to learn—an unexpected lesson at a most unlikely time, and from such a gentle teacher."

But in order for this process to be set in motion, doctors and nurses—in fact, all professional care partners—must be willing to learn new behaviors. They must learn ways to share their feelings and to expose their pain. And the most difficult part of all, they must be willing to be ministered to by others.

138

Here is where there is most resistance to change. This is where "caring" is most out of control—and where "receiving" is most needed. It is here where "giving out" and "giving up"—commonly known in the professional world as "burnout"—is most common.

"BURNOUT": IT'S NOT INEVITABLE

The high incidence of "burnout" among health professionals is not surprising. Doctors strapped with governmental and administrative contraints feel they no longer have control over how patient care is provided. Administrators struggling to stay financially afloat feel powerless to create the centers of healing they had once envisioned. Nurses caught between the demands of doctors and the needs of patients feel exploited and stuck. Everyone, up and down the line, feels that giving care has become more of an ordeal than a privilege.

Their work is hard, and decisions, when made alone, are isolating. For many, this leads to depleted energy and lack of emotional involvement in their work. Some adjust, resigning themselves to the growing conviction that things will never get better. Some deaden themselves to everyone and everything around them. Others exit from the "helping professions" altogether.

But psychologists have discovered that much of this depletion of energy is directly due to what is known as keeping a "professional distance." When professionals deny or minimize their feelings concerning their work, they hold in a great deal of energy and are left feeling drained by this effort. So it stands to reason that one of the first defenses against "burnout" is to begin to find appropriate ways to express feelings.

If this is not done, everyone suffers. One coping strategy that professionals use to minimize their feelings is to belittle or minimize patients. How often we hear staff referring to patients by their illnesses rather than their names."We have a gall bladder in 301 today, an 'appy' in 306, and lots of hernias." When patients are called by name, the same patronizing attitude can persist. "Sally in Room 101 is as cute as a button, a real little doll." Mrs. Jones, in fact, is 70 years old.

Yet health professionals hold firmly to the belief that they must defend themselves emotionally in order to do their jobs. This couldn't be further from the truth. There are other ways that are more healthy for the professional and for everyone involved. One East Coast obstetrician I know was able to expose his true feelings of grief, fear and vulnerability. And through his courage he was able to bring himself and others through the aftermath of a sudden tragedy—the death of a young woman in childbirth—free of bitterness, guilt and recriminations.

During labor, this doctor's patient, a healthy woman with a normal 9-month pregnancy, developed an amniotic fluid embolism, a rare condition which releases highly toxic fluid into the blood stream. It sent the mother-to-be into convulsions and cardiac arrest. She died in labor. Her baby was born dead.

The grief of the family was matched by the grief of the obstetrical office staff—and by the special agony of the doctor. But where most doctors would have minimized their pain or suffered in silence, alone and isolated, this doctor chose another way. He called in a nurse experienced in working with families following neonatal death to work with him and his staff. And he went directly to the home of the grieving family to talk with them. *In other words, he placed himself within their grieving circle.*

Together they explored how they felt about the death —their sense of loss, their rage, their temptation to lash out, their nagging feelings of "if only . . ." And by the end of their time together, they were able to say to each other, "It was not your fault."

So, in fact, the real task for professionals, and the one most healthy for us all, is to learn how to experience our emotions. We must discover that it is possible to experience feelings without being dominated by them, that we can show emotion and still retain composure and competence for the tasks we need to do. And that expressing emotions is important for *our* health as well as for the health of others.

Moreover, patients and family members appreciate and respect staff who can risk being human, can risk showing feelings. A family I worked with respected the training and professionalism of their mother's neurologist. They knew his technical know-how were vital for the competent handling of their mother's debilitating stroke. Yet, they never respected this doctor more than when he could talk to them with tears streaming down his cheeks. Measured against all the knowledge he possessed, all the experience he brought to bear, his depth of feeling increased his stature more than anything else he could have offered them at that moment of need.

Moreover, the emotional bonding this creates is long lasting. At Planetree, former patients come back on the unit to visit nurses they felt were emotionally present for them. If they are hospitalized in another city, they often call back to ask questions of their Planetree nurse. This is what makes nursing worth it all.

One physical therapist who served as a care partner in another hospital said this: "I'll probably never see that patient or his family again. But every time I walk into his old room, I'll remember the laughter, the tears. I'll remember what we did and how good it felt. That memory is what will sustain me and get me through the hard times."

RECEIVING HELP

The second defense against "burnout" is some well-chosen self-indulgence—not just out on the golf course, *but within the hospital setting itself.* In fact, the hospital is where it can count the most because this is where disillusion and discontent with one's work obviously breed and fester.

If only professionals could see that the beginning of the way back is to be kinder to themselves. But few do. When they are encouraged to receive, even from themselves, they feel uncomfortable. Just try to help a nurse. Try to compliment a social worker. As a grateful family member, try to offer a tired surgeon a hot cup of tea. What happens is usually this: They stammer, squirm, give excuses, and vanish from the room as soon as possible.

When Planetree first introduced masseurs and body workers on the unit, its nurses readily recommended their patients for these services, but consistently rejected neck and shoulder massages for themselves. They even admitted that the only nurses who took any kind of break were the smokers, who slipped guiltily into the nurses' lounge for quick cigarettes, then hurried back to their "busy" schedules.

I've sometimes asked health professionals why, when they so obviously need it (and in most cases privately want it), they steadfastly refuse to allow themselves these moments of reprieve. Their answers, while often veiled, suggest deep and complex processes at work, clearly different for every individual. But I note one common thread running through their replies. There are risks involved in receiving help. It's hard to share power, to give up control. At some deep level of our consciousness, being "busy" translates into "being important"—into being in control.

Dr. Paul Brenner, a California physician and author, often lectures on what he calls "the various stages of a healer." In the first stage, a person declares that he or she is going to be a healer, a health professional. This often occurs, Dr. Brenner has discovered, after an early childhood experience with death.

The second stage begins when the young person is entering professional training and ends when he or she has earned the necessary credentials to practice—has become an M.D., a social worker, a nurse, a minister, or whatever. At that point, the attitude toward patients is, according to Brenner, a little like that of Allstate Insurance. "Put yourself in my hands and I'll take care of you."

Brenner uses himself as an example. "After 28 years of school without a break, I knew that I knew exactly how to take care of you. I firmly believed that I was not only well trained, but anything that happened before my training had to be archaic." Today he cautions against second-stage healers with this attitude. "These people can be dangerous, because they need so badly to be in control."

Unfortunately, many health professionals, he reports, remain in stage two. In this stage, a professional rarely accepts help from a patient or anyone else, because he or she does not want to admit that help is needed. And in "stage two" healing, the professional thinks he or she is responsible for everything.

143

Dr. Brenner says the way into stage three occurs when the doctor, nurse, minister realizes that the patient has a great deal to do with the success of the treatment. This usually happens at the point when the healer recognizes the importance of his or her relationship with the patient.

Dr. Brenner's most important learning experience, and the area most health professionals still must explore, occurred in stage four. During this period in his personal/professional odyssey, Dr. Brenner was working with terminally ill patients. These patients were very sick, indeed sick enough to tell Dr. Brenner their life stories, to show all their "honesty cards."

"When these patients would begin to open up their souls to me, I could see so much," Brenner was later to tell lecture audiences. "Not only the radiance in the person, but the radiance in me. It was just as if these patients were healing me, Paul Brenner, of my wounds."

Dr. Brenner makes clear that this stage must be experienced on a "heart level." It can't happen when the health professional maintains emotional distance or remains in control. "When you meet on a heart level," he explains, "there is a mutual healing." In a relationship based on respect and equality, the professional can be healed by the "healee." "It's all in both giving and receiving."

So what keeps healers from moving into the latter and more rewarding stages of their professions? I believe it has to do with the fear of being vulnerable. At the deepest layer of our being, professionals translate receiving help into being vulnerable. And the notion of invulnerability is a highly cherished illusion in medical circles, one that we are particularly loath to give up. But unless we do, our relationships with ourselves and with patients and families will remain out of balance—and thus, less than optimal.

SHARING THE PAIN

Henri Nouwen, author of *The Wounded Healer*, tells a story from the Talmud which relates to this idea and to the essence of care partnering. When the people cried out for a healer, they were told, to their surprise, that when he came he would be poor and covered with bandages. Only through sharing in their pain, they learned, could he know their pain.

But before he could minister to their wounds, he would need to minister to his own. So, too, do modern day professionals. So do care partners. In fact, the story of the "wounded healer" is the story of care partnering, a type of care where professionals as healers must take care of themselves so they'll be ready to take care of others when called upon. They must share in the pain—so they can share in the recovery as well.

INSTITUTIONS THAT ENCOURAGE GROWTH

As the ambulance drove up to the front entrance of Beaumont, Katherine remembered the first time she'd come to this place. At first, she'd put off starting the search for a nursing home for John. All the old stereotypes kept thrusting themselves upon her. At unexpected times, their cruel images would suddenly rush through her head like fast edits in a grotesque horror film.

Patients staring into space.

Patients lying in feces.

Patients covered with bed sores.

But another part of her stubbornly clung to hope. A nursing home didn't have to be that way. There were good ones out there. It was just up to her to find one. She should write down the things she wanted for her father, even some that seemed impossible, and then try her best to get them. After all, if she didn't know what she was looking for, how would she know when she'd found it?

The day she found it, the first thing she noticed about Beaumont was its color and fresh smell. The front lounge was painted yellow. It felt warm and inviting—as if the sun were shining indoors. The air was pure, no odors of yesterday's meatloaf or today's unattended urine.

She noticed the flurry of activity. Some residents were hanging up Christmas cards, some talking at small tables, others listening to music. Behind them on the wall was a sea of photographs, displaying children and grandchildren of residents and staff. And all around them were young people—volunteers, it seemed, pushing wheelchairs and passing out juice.

But what she noticed most were the faces of the people. No glassy-eyed patients overmedicated with tranquilizers. No staff wearied by the routine of nursing home life. The place felt alive.

But if we're to have healers still enthused about their work, we must have institutions that encourage this. We must have organizational structures that urge them to be open about their feelings, that support their healing and their renewal process. Some progressive hospitals and nursing homes are establishing places where staff can share their feelings and receive support. But much more needs to be done. I want to see institutions that actively encourage psychological and spiritual growth among staff, institutions that place value on personal renewal. Why can't those of us working in hospitals have regular massages made available to us, and be given the time to receive them? Why can't we have exercise classes, hatha yoga, deep relaxation and meditation classes right on our premises? Why can't chapels and meditation rooms be open to us as well as to families in crisis? If corporations and businesses, looking for cost-saving ways to achieve higher productivity, can offer classes to exercise bodies and build "quiet rooms" to clear and replenish minds, why not our health care institutions?

Or, if physical places can't be set aside, why not blocks of time? At Planetree, I have suggested that for five minutes at the beginning of each shift, the entire unit—patients, family members and staff—observe an uninterrupted period of quiet together. During this time, the unit doors would be closed to outsiders, no buzzers would ring, no medications delivered. Except in a medical emergency, everyone would honor everyone else's need for silence.

RECEIVING HELP FROM THE "HELPEES"

If "healer, heal thyself" is a precondition of the care partner philosophy, so also is its logical complement: the requirement that patients and families find creative ways to "give to the giver." I'm talking about ways to express appreciation that transcend the traditional box of chocolates or the ritual basket of fruit. Curiously enough, this idea has rarely occurred to most people. Or, if it has, they've rejected it. After all, they're paying the bill. That should take care of their end of the bargain.

But, in fact, it doesn't—not in ways that heal. When I'm assisting a team in preparing a care partner agreement, I always ask, "How will the professional on the team get a break?" There are many kinds of breaks. The break a L.V.N. confers on herself is one kind. The break conferred by the patient or family is another—and often a more effective— kind. "How can you use your special, unique talents," I ask the patient or family member, "to give creatively to the L.V.N., R.N., social worker in the triad?" A care partner agreement

147

should always include ways—uniquely individualized ways—for the "helpee" to help the "helper."

In American Indian tradition, an offering from the heart is always given to the medicine man before a sacred healing ceremony is begun. When I asked Red Hawk, a Karuk medicine man from Northern California, about this custom, he said this: "When a person gives from the heart, he opens his heart to receive the healing. It's part of the preparation."

I've noticed this same phenomenon within the many care partnerships I've witnessed. When a gift comes from the heart, it almost always brings some sort of healing for patient as well as professional. And the source of this energy is almost always love and creativity.

Moreover, I've observed another dynamic at work—the resemblance of creativity to play. Studies of peak performers show that the secret of these people's success is their ability to become absorbed in their work in the same way that children become absorbed in play. While such individuals are achieving at amazingly high levels, they remain focused and relaxed. Their work is their play, and vice versa. Such a finding has a large implication for those dealing with patient illness *and* health professional "burnout." The encouragement of creativity through the opportunity to work with novelty can heal our unhealthy bodies and our unhealthy work environments as well.

The possibilities for creative giving are endless. They can be simple or complicated, expensive or completely free of charge. Each one is distinctly different from the other. The main requirement is that each gift reflect the talents, interest and personality of the giver *and* its recipient.

At Planetree, a patient derived great pleasure and healing energy from designing and printing a plaque for her nurse. Written in finely detailed calligraphy and suitable for framing, it said, "For care and comfort and heartfelt thanks." At the bottom she wrote her name, the name of her nurse, and the date of her hospital confinement.

Recently a former Planetree patient invited four of his nurses to a dinner party at Act IV, a lovely San Francisco restaurant. "Only my finances," he said, "kept me from inviting the entire staff."

At other hospitals, I've heard other stories. One elderly patient packed her suitcase with nightgown, bed jacket, camera and film. Over the course of her confinement, following a total hip replacement, she chronicled the work of her physical therapist. As the therapist worked on her, she worked on the therapist. And upon her discharge two weeks later, she presented her healer with a photo album entitled, "Two Weeks in the Life of a Dedicated Therapist: With Appreciation From a Grateful Patient."

One patient wrote out the names of each aide who had been especially thoughtful to him. Then he sent out spies to find out each one's favorite perfume. On his discharge day, when his family brought him his clothes, they also brought small bottles of Chanel No. 5, Estee Lauder and Yves Saint Laurent. These he presented to his aides, one by one, letting the surprise gift say what he could not.

The gifts must not only be specific and individualized, they must spark the enthusiasm of the giver. This personal interest and involvement is the ingredient that moves patients from sickness to health. This is the miracle drug available without prescription.

I know a patient who, when she found her anesthesiologist was from Kentucky, promptly ordered him a Kentucky ham. Another patient, a musician who had just given birth, wrote an I.O.U. to her obstetrician's wife, offering to sing at a birthday party the wife had planned for her husband. In still another case, a pediatrician was surprised by a birthday party planned, with the help of his receptionist, by his young patients and their grateful parents.

Appreciation can be expressed privately with a word or a hug—or it can be announced publicly. I know one family who wrote the supervisor of the respiratory therapist they had worked with to express their high regard for the quality of his work. They made copies for all important members of the hospital staff and asked that the letter be included in the therapist's personnel file. I know a daughter-in-law who wrote to the Commissioner of her state's Department of Health to commend a nursing home administrator for her outstanding leadership and direction. A copy went to the nursing home and one to the nursing home's corporate office.

Patients, on the suggestion of receptionists or librarians, have purchased needed and valued medical books for their doctors, nurses, or their hospital's library. Inside the covers they've written personally chosen inscriptions. One nurse told me her favorite gift was a birthday card she'd received from a former cardiac patient. The card came not on *her* birthday, but on *his*. He wrote, "Because of you, I'm alive to celebrate this day."

I know a church group which organized a care program for a private duty nurse who was caring for a member of their congregation. Each day someone from the church brought in lunch for the nurse, steeped her tea, and stood in for her while she went out for a breath of fresh air. The idea was to focus love and attention on this particular caregiver. This nurse was caring for their friend, so they would care for this nurse.

The beauty of the care partner program is that it identifies one person or a small group of persons on which the patient or family member can focus. I've known of many families who have had good experiences in hospitals, but have had no realistic way to thank all the nurses, aides, orderlies and technicians on three different shifts. Because of the overwhelming numbers, the "thank you's" were never sent. And those who should have received them never knew how much they were appreciated.

"This is your home now," said the nurse, leading Katherine and her father into the room assigned to John. Katherine looked around. A pleasant room. The touches of red in the wallpaper and bedspread were picked up by two large poinsettia plants, brought in for the holidays. Aunt Dorothy had arrived before them. Her prisms, already at the window, cast moving flecks of amber around the room, their radiance mixing and mingling with the scarlet of the flowers.

Katherine looked at her father, but he didn't look back. His eyes were still covered with patches, his face a mask.

"Maybe you should think about removing the patches, at least for part of the day," the nurse said as if reading Katherine's thought. Then she turned directly to John. "It seems to me, Mr. McGuire, if you're to come out of this coma and live, maybe some visual stimulation would help." As she left the room, she said to Katherine, "Think about it."

Eyes are the windows to the soul. Katherine remembered the old saying and wondered if she really wanted to do this, wanted to see what she might find. She studied the squares of white gauze and paper tape that covered her father's eye sockets. Then, carefully, hesitantly, she lifted them off.

She looked down into her father's open eyes. The same brown irises flecked with gold. The same sandy lashes. At that moment, he looked up at her.

In her excitement she wanted to call the nurse, to tell her what

151

had happened. She wanted to let her know how much she appreciated this sign of special concern for her dad.

But suddenly Katherine was summoned to the office. And in her hurry, she let the moment pass.

PART II: BUILDING SUPPORT FROM
WITHIN AND WITHOUT

Katherine had almost forgotten the special smells and textures of her mother's old family home—the home of the Burtons' side of the family since Civil War days. Old wood and metal objects, worn by the handling of many hands. Musty fabrics holding on to time. They filled the rooms with an almost tangible presence, as if the ghosts of four generations were everywhere around her.

She'd also forgotten how her mother, at times like these, reverted to her Southern past. The whole family was gathered together—everyone, that is, except John, who still lay silent in the nursing home ten miles away.

"It's time we had some plain grub," Agnes declared from the kitchen. "That hospital food's been killing us. We need some turnip greens, corn bread and black-eyed peas." It was customary to eat black-eyed peas for good luck on New Year's Day. They were just early by two days.

"Cornbread made from Martha White Corn Meal!" Katherine called out from the pantry. "That's one thing I haven't forgotten."

At dinner, she regaled her family with tales of how her "Yankee" friends made cornbread. "They use sugar. Can you imagine?"

"And I bet you can't even get turnip greens out there."

"You can, but only from garbage cans."

Although the still figure alone in the nursing home was never far from their minds, this brief respite from responsibility helped to loosen the knots of anxiety weighing on their spirits and isolating them from one another. As they laughed at the vagaries of life outside the South, they found themselves drawing together as a family, girding themselves for what lay ahead.

This family was adopting an age-old survival tactic. In the face of serious illness of a loved one, it was grasping the nearest remedy at hand—a home-cooked meal and a "Yankee joke." But the precise nature of the remedy wasn't important. Whatever worked was O.K. A good cry with friends, an evening around the fire, a matinee and lunch downtown would have been just as good. The point is that a little self-indulgence is absolutely essential, not only for the close relatives and friends doing the all-night vigils, but for those feeling guilty about *not* doing them.

In the care partner program, family members, like health professionals, learn how to give to themselves. One man I know reinstated a meditation practice he had started years before his wife's illness. That enabled him to concentrate his energy on being in the hospital for long stretches. Another friend indulged herself by refusing to comply with social pressures that might add stress to her life. She declined all dinner invitations or social engagements if she was expected to dress up, be on time, or make small talk. She chose to devote all her energies to coping with the stresses of the hospital where her brother lay ill.

For these people, the idea was to feel renewed despite being in the hospital virtually all the time. For others, the best strategy is to get away from the hospital. Sometimes I recommend a long walk or a visit to the hairdresser. Do something purely hedonistic, I tell people. A shopping spree perhaps? Anything—*anything at all*—to introduce everyday incentives and an element of normalcy into an otherwise abnormal situation.

A friend called me recently to say he'd set up a care partner program while caring for two hospitalized parents in another part of the state. Since they were in separate institutions, the demand on his time and energy was great. So outside the hospital he chose to do only those things that would replenish him. He let household chores go undone; he didn't worry about cooking, choosing to dine out at restaurants instead. He set up an exercise program of swimming and jogging, strictly adhering to it even though it cut into his hospital visits. Most important, he called his wife and asked her to drop everything and come to him. "I need you," he was able to say.

TAKING THE RISK OF ASKING

More and more people today are taking these risks. Like the wounded healer, they are sharing their pain, asking for what they need. A father, through his local newspaper, requested cards for his five-year-old son in a coma. In less than a week, the response came—books, stuffed animals, 150 cards and letters, and $500 in cash.

A young mother with cancer prepared a list of things her friends could do to lend a hand to her family during her hospital stays. Here are a few.

"Cook a dinner for my family, but offer a choice of two courses. One week we got tuna noodle casserole four nights in a row from well-meaning friends! Also, bring the food in disposable containers or marked pots. If I can't return your casserole, I will cry at my powerlessness and confusion.

Help my children attend birthday parties by bringing some pre-wrapped children's birthday party gifts to our home for future use.

Offer to run two meaningless errands a week for our family. The small stuff—like no hair ribbons, or cologne, or clean suits—fall by the wayside otherwise.

Encourage your husband to come over to visit my husband in the evenings. One of the greatest gifts I have is my husband; yet my illness has eliminated many of his pleasures."

Here was a *patient* setting up a support network for her *family*, a variation on what we've been discussing, but a perfect example of simultaneously giving and receiving. Wendy Bergren's ideas, published under the title "Mom is Very Sick—Here's How to Help," have guided not only her friends but thousands of other people across the country who want to be a "help" not a "hindrance."

Networks of friends are equated by Dennis Jaffe and Cynthia Scott to sunglasses filtering out the harsh glare that occasionally comes into our personal and professional lives. Their metaphor, used in their book *From Burnout to Balance*, is particularly apt in this context. While experiencing the stress of hospital life, we should use our friends and colleagues as sunglasses to shield us from the increased pressures brought on by crisis. They can, in the most literal sense, be good medicine.

WHAT ARE FRIENDS FOR?

Reverend Bingham met Katherine in the hall of the nursing home and walked her to a quiet place. A man in his forties with dark, closely cropped hair, he had deep-set, searching blue eyes which dominated his face. Katherine fixed those eyes with her own, as she described what she needed.

"The family's so tired, I'm not sure we're going to last without some help. All kinds of people come to see Dad and ask if they can do something. They mean well, but most of the time they just wear us out."

"Have you thought how they could help?"

Katherine's palms had turned moist. Before starting to speak, she'd had no idea how hard it would be for her to ask directly for what she wanted.

"Well, as a matter of fact I have," she began weakly. "We could use a coordinator, one person to check with us each day to see what we need." Having said that, she found herself warming to her subject. "For instance, what we could use right now is sitters during the evening meal. We need to eat together at home—to get our strength back and meet and plan as a family. But we'd rather not leave Dad alone. If a coordinator could schedule people to come from 6 to 8 each evening, I think they might enjoy doing something useful and we'd get some relief."

Katherine was shocked at what she'd just asked. She'd always been taught to be "nice," even if that included being dishonest. It was the Southern way, the acceptable way for women to push for what they wanted without seeming "pushy." So now it was hard to speak simply and straightforwardly, not to resort to elaborate diplomacy and indirection.

Sweaty palms, though understandable, weren't necessary. When people are asked to become "givers," they are usually flattered. When they're given specific guidelines on how to give most effectively, they're reassured. When they're given a guilt-free opportunity to say "no" if they can't meet requests, they're grateful. During the McGuires' story, there occurred many variations on this theme. When direct requests were carefully structured, they worked. When interactions were marked by mutual giving and receiving, they not only worked—they blossomed.

The tall, rawboned man rounded the door with a long, swinging gait and introduced himself in the slow drawl of the rural South. "I'm Clarence Mayberry, your father's barber. I just heard you were looking for someone to help." He thrust out his hand to her. It was large like a logger's, but with sensitive fingers more like an artist's.

157

He listened quietly to Katherine's standard talk—tips on what the sitters should watch out for and what they might do with John during the dinner hour. Since this was his first time to "sit," she reassured him, "I won't be long."

"Don't worry, Ma'am, take as long as you need. I have nothing I'd rather do than be here." As he spoke, he wandered around the room looking at the posters, chuckling at the messages written on them. Peering closely at a photo of John, he remarked, "Shoulda come in and seen me before that one."

"How long have you known Dad?"

"Oh, since back in the 1950s, twenty-five or thirty years, I guess."

"What did you two talk about all that time?"

"He liked to talk about golf, of course, and different sports. He was always telling me about you out in California and about Teddy. Showed me pictures of his grandchildren. Of course, I like to read the funny papers and he did, too. We both thought Dagwood ought to run Blondie off."

Katherine was putting some things away, preparing to leave, when her eye lit on the razor she used each day to shave her father. "This is the first time I've ever shaved anyone," she said talking to the pro. "How do you think he looks?"

"Looks like you're doing just fine—but, you'll excuse me, Ma'am, when I walked in I couldn't help noticing a spot you missed. He likes a close shave. And he wants his hair short and neat. 'Get 'er close,' he always says."

"Do you think it looks a little long now?"

"Longer than he wears it." Clarence came over to John's bed, giving his hair a quick scrutiny. "Tell you what. How about if I get my scissors out of the car and cut it for him, just like he likes it."

"After you've cut hair all day? Isn't that too much?"

"It's not hard to do something for someone you like. It's not hard at all."

A clergyman I knew once told me about an unusual family he'd dealt with who were entirely open and direct about the help they needed during a hospital crisis. "It was refreshing," he said. "With some families, I feel I have to be a mind reader, trying to guess what they want. That family, by letting me know straight out what I could do for them, gave me a chance to minister in ways that are rarely open to me."

When I talked with a doctor and his wife who had been chosen to serve on a care partner team, they said something similar about their experience. In fact they reported that the help they received from the family was more than they felt they gave. "We were having a problem with one of our children at the time, and somehow this experience helped to clear that up. Maybe it was getting a better perspective on our situation, seeing the larger picture through exposure to a life and death struggle. Yes, we gained from the program."

But even when we know the givers stand to benefit, we still hesitate. Why? Barbara, a single mother, needed at least one person who loved her to support her during her pregnancy and confinement. So she invited *ten* people to serve on her "birthing team." For six months she made requests of them. Each one responded when the request was possible and said "no" when it was not. In small clusters they went on hospital tours, watched childbirth movies, attended classes where they squatted on their haunches and took deep breaths from their abdomens. Finally, when the labor began, the ten of them showed up at the hospital bearing flowers, tape recorder and music, fruit juice—ready for the day's work.

When I asked Barbara how she got the courage to ask so many people to do so many things for her, she admitted that two years earlier she couldn't have asked. "I didn't believe that people would do things for me. I wouldn't have dared ask. I guess I just didn't feel worthy. Now I do."

REJECTION ANXIETY: THE UNIVERSAL FEAR

Teddy, Katherine's brother, spoke first. "Mother and I have been talking it over, and we think the 'sitting' has to stop."
"What do you mean?" Katherine asked.
"No more sitters," Agnes said with a tone of finality.
"Why not?"
"For a week now, people have come through for us. But we can't keep asking," Teddy said. "The town'll begin to say, if they need sitters, they should pay for them."
"Some of the younger women have children at home," interrupted Agnes. "They shouldn't be coming out at dinner time, just to help us out."
"Shouldn't that be their decision?" Katherine blurted out. "How can we know how they feel? Maybe people who love Dad and our family need a way to show us?"
"Yeah, but how would we feel if they started turning us down."

"What if I get turned down?" It's a nagging question that plagues most of us when we contemplate asking for help. Hearing how the people of a small Southern town turned out for "sitting," one is apt to reply, "Maybe it could happen in a place like that, where everybody knows everyone else. But in New York? In Chicago? Not likely."

And on hearing a story like Barbara's, one's skepticism tends to mount. "That's well and good for people who live in California and don't have entrenched traditions. They're more willing to try something strange."

But, in fact, no matter where people live or what circumstances they're dealing with, they're only too ready to believe, "My friends would never come through like that for me."

I wanted to test the widespread theory that most people

shun requests from those in medical crisis. So I searched for examples of families in large urban centers who had experienced such rejections. I queried medical social workers, chaplains, psychologists, nurses in hospitals and in home care settings throughout the San Francisco Bay Area. I could find no examples.

To explain why, one psychotherapist offered this hypothetical situation: "Suppose I'm walking through a supermarket and a stranger stops me and says she's recovering from back surgery. She asks me to lift a bag of dog food into her cart. Of course I'll do it. Who wouldn't? When people who are ill or in pain tell you exactly what they need and let you know your help is important to them, you'll almost always respond. In fact, you'll usually go way beyond what's asked of you."

Granted, we all enjoy playing supermarket samaritan if it doesn't take more than five minutes. We may even be able to sustain that good feeling for a period of days or weeks, when a close friend or relative needs us. But how long we would cheerfully play that role if it were indefinitely extended is debatable. When we hear stories of individuals like Mother Teresa, we ask ourselves guiltily, "Would I be capable of that?" And we suspect not.

Knowing that about ourselves—that pure altruism is normally of limited duration—and suspecting that others have a similar finite capacity for "good works," we struggle with rejection anxiety. We know all too well the dark places in the human psyche— because they exist in our own.

But in striving to be realistic about "human nature," we often distort reality. Guarding against a feared rebuff, we bring on one that was never intended. Or, by avoiding a direct statement of what we need, we force people to guess what's on our minds—and then, when they guess wrong, take *that* as rejection.

161

EDITH: Look, I'm your next door neighbor, your best friend. Please tell me what you need?

MILDRED: Listen, I know how busy you are. Don't worry with me. *(Why can't she see what I need. I need the same help I gave her sister when she was sick last year.)*

EDITH: But if I knew what would help you, I'd do it.

MILDRED: *(She must be blind. She knows I don't drive. She knows how nervous I am to take the bus, how scared I am of this place and everything that's happening to Bill.)* Honestly, I can't think of a thing.

EDITH: But without some hint from you, there's not much I can really do.

MILDRED: That's all right. Don't worry about it. *(I knew all along she didn't care.)*

The problem, then, is not so much that those in need are being rejected, but that they are setting things up so they will be. Rollo May, who helped pioneer the humanistic psychology movement, writes in his classic text *The Meaning of Anxiety* that anxiety and fear arise when the infant becomes apprehensive over possible disapproval from the significant people in his life, usually the mother. When the infant senses a real or imagined lack of interest on the part of the mother—and this is apt to happen to all babies at some time or other—he may internalize that response and define himself as unlovable. Because of these early precognitive experiences, any hint of indifference or criticism by others later in life may trigger this primitive fear of rejection and abandonment. Thus, according to May, the child, and later the adult, seeking to ensure survival, learns to tailor his behavior to avoid rejection.

More recently, Jordan and Margaret Paul, psychotherapists and co-authors of the popular book *Do I Have to Give Up Me to Be Loved by You?* say that virtually everyone experiences some doubts and insecurities about adequacy and lovability. Most people learn ways to avoid or rationalize signs of rejection, even the mildest reprimand from a boss or the subtlest slight at a party. But avoidance becomes even more intense when our most deeply felt emotions are on the line.

"The situation we all fear the most because it hurts the most," they write, "is the loss of love." For some of us, this fear creates such all-consuming anxiety that we will do anything—sacrifice anything—to protect against it. Even though we want intimacy, many of us would rather give up the opportunity for love than suffer the pain of losing love.

Rollo May and the Pauls have neatly identified the dynamics we are concerned with here. Because of our extreme fear of rejection from others, we tend to set things up so that we are never in a position to be refused. By fending off others' love before they can refuse to give it, we beat them to the punch. We reject ourselves before they have a chance to do it for us.

But the price we pay is profound. We come to believe that we are unworthy of love. And this leads to the final step in this cruel logic—the conviction that others can never love us in the ways we need and want.

SUPPORT: IT'S REALLY THERE FOR THE ASKING

They gathered in the activity room. This was where meetings at the nursing home were usually held. People pulled their metal folding chairs into a circle on the bare parquet floor, just cleared after exercise class. Around them were an old upright piano, a small refrigerator, and a long formica counter with an electric coffee maker at one end.

Agnes sat, tense and apprehensive, on the edge of her chair. She wasn't sure she wanted to be at this meeting. They'd called it a "planning session" to talk about John's *"treatment plan."* She wasn't sure what that was supposed to be. A kind of get-together, she supposed, of the family, the administrator, the director of nursing, the physical therapist, the speech therapist, the nutritionist, the social worker—all of them figuring out how to *"individualize"* John's care and get everyone doing things for him.

Like seeing that he got moved every day. Seeing that his teeth got cleaned. Seeing that he heard his ballgame scores.

It seemed pretty far-fetched to Agnes. What she was wondering was if she'd be expected to keep things up the way Katherine, Sarah and Dorothy had—after they'd gone home to their families and the whole job was left on her shoulders.

Abruptly breaking her silence, she announced to the circle, "I won't be able to be here every day, all day long, the way the others have."

The administrator, moving quickly to take advantage of this opening, replied, "When you feel tired, you stay home and get the rest you need. We'll take care of John. But when you want to come, just know that you'll be welcome any time, day or night. We have no visiting hours here."

"But that's just it," said Agnes, still clinging to her doubts. "I never know if I can get here. I don't drive when it's snowing anymore. It makes me too nervous."

"If the roads are icy and you really want to be here, we'll find you a ride," the administrator assured her. "We have an arrangement with the National Guard to help us in these situations. The main thing is for you to know we're here to help you as well as your husband."

Agnes moved back in her chair. The taut muscles at the back of her neck had begun to relax a little. And the pain in her back had started to fade.

The members of the care partner triad can help themselves and help each other. But sometimes it's necessary to supplement that help from the outside. Is such support really there for the asking? I believe it is.

In most hospitals and nursing homes, there are services designed to help families right on the premises. For example, the social service unit will link up families with meals, transportation, financial assistance, counseling and self-help groups. Family support groups may be operating right in the institution. For out-of-town relatives of acute care patients, access to guest rooms is sometimes offered at reduced rates in or near the hospital.

One excellent example of hospital-based support is the "Anderson Network," located at the M.D. Anderson Hospital and Tumor Institute, a University of Texas System Cancer Center in Houston. Prior to admission or during their hospitalization, cancer patients or their families can request help and support from a network of over 100 former cancer patients.

At the University of Alabama in Birmingham, through a program called "Touch," former patients join inpatients and family members in a weekly support group to talk about treatment methods and the hospital experience.

Across the country through programs like "Heart-to-Heart," and "Reach-to-Recovery," former patients visit and support hospitalized patients recovering from heart attacks, mastectomies, or other medical traumas.

Out in the community, services abound. At Century Village, a retirement community in Deerfield, Florida, two residents became concerned about friends and neighbors who went into hospitals without proper support. So they created support. Through a program called "We Care," resident volunteers are matched with patients, and sometimes with spouses and families of patients. Often the support provided during the hospitalization continues after the patients are discharged home. The Redwoods Retirement Community in Mill Valley, California, has a similar program called "Care and Share," where residents give and receive help from one another.

For families facing the responsibility of caregiving for the terminally ill, hospice organizations are also prepared to serve caregiver as well as patient and to serve within the institution as well as outside its walls.

A San Francisco man in his nineties was dying of cancer. His caregiver was his wife, a woman of 82. The hospice team summoned to help soon realized that she needed as much help as he did. Their first move was to contact the couple's local church and the closest senior center and to set up a group of sitters to relieve the wife *on a regular basis*. That way she knew that on specific days she could *count* on going out to lunch at a nearby senior center. And during certain hours she could *plan* on taking a nap at home.

When the patient came home, hospice supplied the basic framework for the care program by providing a nurse and two home health aides to do bathing, laundry and meals. Along with the sitters were other services set up by the hospice staff, but provided by volunteers—art and music therapy, massage for both patient and wife, recreation activities supplied by a local center for the handicapped. Apart from a few church members, the various components of this care team had little or no acquaintance with one another and had never known the family until the husband became ill.

By designing the care program along these lines, the hospice team brought together services already in place within the community. In areas where no formal services existed, it identified individuals willing to help. And by melding these components together, it created a single, integrated support system.

Something like this, though perhaps less extensive, is often needed to restore both family and hospital staff during long and very difficult hospitalizations. And I'm convinced that those who look for it or ask for it can find it right in their midst.

ORGANIZATIONS—THE BEST SOURCE OF ORGANIZED SUPPORT

Her friends called her "The General." A retired nurse with a talent for taking charge. Madeline knew how to organize people and get things done. Within days after members of Katherine's California church heard of her departure to Tennessee—and why—they mobilized under Madeline's leadership to support Katherine's husband, Doug, and their two young sons.

Madeline started out by interviewing Doug and the boys separately, asking each what kind of meals he liked, what time he was used to eating, where he needed to be driven each day (school? dentist appointments? after-school sports?) and when. By the following day, she had given them a chart with the menu for the following week written on it and the name of the scheduled chef (a different church member for each day) noted by each meal. Bits of additional information were jotted beside each item.

"Hold the mushrooms."

"Absolutely no artichokes."

All Doug and the boys had to do was return the empty dishes to the church on Sundays. The boys had promptly dubbed Madeline's project "OPERATION SUPERBOWL."

The most valuable aspect of working through organizations is the helping network they already have in place.

Organizations have names, headquarters, phone numbers and usually systems ready to go into action. And these groups usually come with long track records. Take organized religion, for example. Religious communities were the original caregivers of the sick, the aged and the poor. With the industrialization of our society, organized religion has turned most of these responsibilities over to government and nonprofit health and social service agencies. But individual churches still see themselves as support systems for their members who are sick or for non-members who specifically ask for their help.

In fact, many churches have the rudiments of a care partner program already functioning. Some merely store sick room supplies, wheelchairs, bed pans and the like. Some offer visitation services. Others have more formal programs for hospitalized patients and their families.

A Protestant program most closely approximating the care partner approach is called the Stephens Ministry. Founded by Kenneth C. Haugh, a pastor and clinical psychologist, this program has trained over 50,000 lay counselors over the past dozen years in over 50 denominations in the United States, Canada, Australia, Germany, the Panama Canal Zone and the Middle East. Along with training in other areas of crisis and need, the Stephens Ministry offers a high level of training to lay people prepared to work with individuals and families experiencing the stress of hospitalization. In the state of Oregon, Stephens Ministers are stationed in many emergency and surgery waiting rooms, where they are directly available to family members.

To be put in touch with someone to serve as a care partner or as support to a care partner team, those interested need only call the Ministry's St. Louis headquarters and ask how to contact the Stephens program closest to their hospital.

The Catholic Church also offers special programs for those suffering grief or loss and those dealing with AIDS and other illnesses. To find out more about these programs, interested parties should call their local parish or diocesan Catholic Charities office.

Most Jewish synogogues have a Chaverah to provide the fellowship and assistance of an extended family when one's natural family lives far away. Within the reform movement there may be "pararabbinics," trained lay counselors similar to the Stephens Ministers, who will visit those in medical crisis.

Finally, all three of these religions sponsor men's and women's groups that support families in need. Through the Catholic Social Services, the Jewish Family and Children's Services, and many Protestant centers, pastoral counseling and therapy are available and provided by professionally trained clinicians.

Those without church affiliation can simply look in the telephone Yellow Pages and call any church or synogogue listed there. I asked a minister I know if a person unknown to his church could call for help and get a meaningful response. "Yes," he said. "All it would take is for the caller to connect with one person in the church who cared enough to set the gears in motion. The rest would quickly follow."

For those who feel secular organizations would be more appropriate for them, the best numbers to call are the local Volunteer Bureau, the nearest branch of the American Red Cross or the American Cancer Society, or whatever group is associated with the illness in question.

SUPPORT FROM STRANGERS

The Beaumont Nursing Home housed a rich collection of personalities who, in their several ways, formed relationships with the

169

McGuires. There was the man in the room next to John's. He was blind, but every day he'd drop by to see how the family was doing. There was the young man in the baseball cap, who regularly reminded the family that he, too, had been in a coma. There were the two black men in wheelchairs who rolled up to the side door to unlock it for Katherine when she visited late at night.

But the two ladies who stood sentinel at the front door were the most consistently attentive. The self-appointed greeters of the nursing home, they knew as much, or more, than the staff about what went on there. They knew whose condition had worsened and whose had improved. They knew who had received visitors that day, what relation they were to the patient, and whether they were from town or from out-of-town.

One of the ladies always had a teddy bear nestled in her lap. "My granddaughter gave me this for Christmas," she would call out to anyone passing through, whether or not they had asked.

The ladies saw it as their responsibility to give the family daily reports on John's visitors and his mail. "Harry Corrigan from down at the garage came in yesterday after you left," one of them would announce brightly. "Wanted you to know your mother's car still needed some more work. And, say, there's something in the mail for your daddy. We already took it down to him."

"Yes," chirped her companion, a tiny meticulously dressed woman with billows of black/grey hair fastened high on her head with a jeweled comb. "We always cheer him up, tell him all the news. He likes to know everything, you know."

Sometimes help comes naturally as part of the everyday course of events. It comes because of the interest and goodwill of the "strangers" around you. What's more, finding these strangers is easier than you may think. Look around in your hospital waiting room or nursing home corridors. You'll usually find others there with problems and needs much like your own. And before you know it, you'll discover yourself forming deep emotional relationships. These relationships aren't based on a shared history, but on the demands of a particular moment in time. I call them "crisis friendships."

A young woman found herself in a hospital waiting room far removed from her home town, waiting to hear news of her critically ill father. Her mother was paralyzed with grief and fear. Responsibility for acting on her family's behalf seemed to rest with her. As the waiting grew longer and she felt her own strength ebbing, she began to reflect, with a hint of panic, that she had no friends in this town to turn to—or at least she didn't think she had.

Who the short, squat little man was, or where he came from, she never knew. She never even knew his name. Yet at the critical moment, when desperation had started to set in, he moved to her side and began to calm her. His wife had chronic pulmonary disease, and he had become a veteran of waiting rooms. He knew how to deal with insurance forms. He knew what to ask doctors and what not to ask. He knew which staff to approach for which equipment. But more important, he knew when to confirm this woman's feelings with reassurances and when to speak unwelcome truths to her.

A few days after they first met outside the ICU, her long vigil still unresolved, he said to her bluntly. "You're losing weight and you look awful. Call your husband and tell him to get up here this weekend." He gave her the name of a nearby motel with a pool and a sauna.

Forty-eight hours later, rested and cheered by the news that her father was out of danger, she looked around to thank her friend, but the crisis had gone and so had he.

SUPPORT FROM THE MIND

I sometimes set up personal support teams which are entirely products of my imagination. With them, there are no limits to what I can ask, and there are never rejections. I can draw upon my personal heroes, famous people who've never heard of me, people too far away or far too busy, people who have been long dead.

In the course of writing this book, I have called together Dr. Paul Brenner, Dr. Bernie Siegel and Norman Cousins, three authors who have written about positivity, creativity and their effects on health; Madeleine L'Engle, who suffered ten years of rejections from every major American publisher before the bulk of her 25 books appeared in print; Anne Lamott, my Marin County neighbor and author of *Hard Laughter*, who makes me laugh and reminds me not to take myself too seriously; and Virginia Hine, author of a favorite book of mine, *Last Letter to the Pebble People*, who died in 1982.

I visualize it all—my invitations, their arrival at my house. They're always on time and always in the best of humor. They gather around my dining room table, eager to help me. I talk to them and they talk to me, always supporting me in the most positive and helpful ways.

Does this sound outlandish? A bit too fanciful for a sensible adult? Perhaps. But actually, there's nothing unusual about it. Just think how good it feels to be around someone you love and admire, someone who in turn respects and cares about you. If such intimates aren't immediately at hand, you can supply them with your mind. Children do it all the time. They conjure up whole troops of imaginary friends and pets. If they can get psychological payoffs from such strategies, why can't we?

HOW MUCH CAN WE ASK?

"Teddy's leaving tomorrow with the only car we have," Katherine told Reverend Bingham on the phone. *"Dad's car was damaged in the accident and Mother's is in the garage. So we're going to be without transportation to and from the nursing home."*

Within an hour, he was back to her. "I've found you a car. Is stick shift all right?"

"Unfortunately, no. Neither Sarah nor I can drive a stick shift." She felt embarrassed and discouraged. It had been a small miracle that the first car had been offered. A second miracle seemed out of the question.

But while the situation seemed hopeless to her, it didn't to the Reverend. "Don't worry," he said cheerfully. "Something'll work out." And something did. Informed of the problem, the owner of the offered car called back and proudly announced he'd made a trade with one of his employees—his 1975 stick shift for the man's 1969 automatic. So the miracle had come full circle. The '69 Chevy not only ran, but she and Sarah could drive it!

How far can we go when asking for help? In an emergency, there should be no limits. Drs. Peter Rosenbaum and John Beebe write in their widely respected textbook *Psychiatric Treatment,* "[When you are] working in an emergency context, [you have] a right to call anyone, however far away, and make unusual demands . . . No one is going to blame [you] for doing everything [you] can do to respond to the emergency."

But what about situations that, technically speaking, are not emergencies? Asking for help under any circumstances can be daunting. You're making yourself vulnerable. Bridge players can understand that. Being vulnerable in bridge poses the danger of a penalty. But it also offers the possibility of a bonus. Go for the bonus. The risk of asking directly for what you want, whether you meet acceptance or rejection, can move you out of helplessness into empowerment. It can propel you out of hopelessness into hope. It can bring you out of isolation into the warmth of human contact.

And, most miraculous of all, it can do the same thing for those who help you. Every player in the game can end up winning.

> MILDRED: I have to admit, I really do need some help. Now that Bill's coming home, he'll have to go back for chemotherapy for the next six weeks. I can't drive and I don't want him riding the bus. Could you drive us to the hospital at 9 on Tuesdays?
>
> EDITH: I can drop you off on the way to work, but I can't bring you home.
>
> MILDRED: Well, I'll see if someone else can do it.
>
> EDITH: Wait a minute. Dorothy and Emily told me they wanted to help. So have John and Isabelle. I've just thought of a way. I'll invite them to my house Friday night and we'll figure out a schedule for you. It's only for six weeks. We can handle that.
>
> MILDRED: Are you sure?
>
> EDITH: Listen, I haven't had any friends over for ages. It'll be a good excuse for a party. Maybe Bill will feel well enough for you both to come over, too.
>
> MILDRED: We'll bring the dip.

Chapter 7

HANDLING CRITICAL CARE

PART I: WHEN THE PATIENT MAY RECOVER

The doctor, there for John's examination, suddenly broke off from his sing-song report. Silently he went over his standard exam again—heart, lungs, temperature, blood pressure. When he'd finished, he stood a moment in thought. Then he circled the bed and walked slowly toward Katherine. In a tone of frank disbelief, he said in a near whisper, "It's just possible he's going to live."

For a split second, her spirits soared. The thought flashed through her mind, why whisper? Why not shout it out—exuberantly! But in another second, she knew the answer.

"Do you mean he may live, but in a coma?"

"Probably. And then again, maybe not. It's hard to tell at this point. Don't get your hopes up. The possibility is very remote."

Whenever there is reason to believe that a patient will live—either fully recovered or seriously impaired—the quality of the care given during the period when he or she hangs in the balance can sometimes make the difference between life and death. Our critical care units, both intensive care and coronary care, should command the highest quality staff, the most concentrated effort, and the most advanced technology of all units in our medical institutions. In most good hospitals today, they do.

But there is an ingredient missing in these specialized units of modern care. To sense what it is, all we need do is experience one and note its effect on patients. Intensive care units are just like they sound—*intense*. There is an urgent quality about them. Decisions must be made quickly and correctly. Space is limited and there is little privacy. Often the entire unit is one large room, with patients not only visible to the nurses, but to other patients as well. Even when there are separate rooms, patients must usually wear devices enabling nurses to continuously monitor vital signs on television screens mounted at their stations. In this kind of environment—where unpredictable intrusions from people and invasive treatments from machines must be endured 24 hours a day—patients tend to adapt the best they can. Many, in order to cope, withdraw emotionally. Some lapse into helplessness, fear, confusion, and sometimes worse.

ONLY IN THE ICU

There is, in fact, a syndrome called "the ICU psychosis." This is where psychologically normal people behave in psychotic ways—hallucinating, hearing voices, becoming violent. This usually occurs only in the ICU. Once the patient is discharged onto other floors, the psychotic behavior typically disappears. The cause of ICU psychosis is not fully known.

Some feel it's an organic reaction to the physical trauma or treatment that brought the patient to the ICU. Some believe it's a psychiatric reaction to the ICU environment itself.

"Sundowning" is yet another condition that occurs more often in intensive settings than anywhere else in the hospital. This is where normally functioning patients exhibit extreme confusion, irritability, bizarre, and/or violent behaviors, but only at night. Patients find it far more difficult to distinguish between night and day in intensive units, where few if any windows give clues to the time of day. The drone of equipment and the glare of lights go on 24 hours nonstop. Activity is incessant and, without proper medical control, so is pain.

If this were not damaging enough, those best able to soothe and comfort patients—close relatives and friends—are forbidden entrance. When visits are allowed, they are only for a few minutes during prearranged hours.

THE MISSING INGREDIENT

What is missing in critical care, then, is the very ingredient that is ordinarily banned—loved ones. The reasons given for the ban are that inexperienced lay people "trying to help" pose too much risk to desperately ill patients trying to recover. And indeed that *could* be the case—if the risk is unmanaged. If visiting is perceived in the traditional way—regarded as a necessary evil to be barely tolerated, rather than a golden opportunity to be carefully utilized—then, of course, family visits will remain unproductive, an inconvenient distraction for staff and perhaps a dangerous drain on patients.

But a care partner program—a very special kind, especially designed for critical care—can meet and overcome virtually all these objections. Indeed, care partners, when

177

properly trained and desensitized, can perform miracles in counteracting the negative effects of intensive care settings.

Here are some examples. To prevent or reduce disorientation, a care partner can bring in clocks and calendars that patients can see from their beds. I know a care partner who gave her patient a pen to mark off each hospital day on his calendar. There he recorded the agenda for each day: the time his doctor would make rounds; the time for his physical therapy; the time of his evening medications; and his time for sleep.

Other things can be done. If the patient is used to reading the morning paper at 7:00, read it to him. If he says prayers at night before bed, say them with him. Familiar love objects (called transition objects by psychologists) make even more sense when a patient is fearful and confused. I know one family who covered three walls of a coronary care room with Spuds McKenzie. Straight from the beer commercial came the patient's favorite mascot on big bright wall posters, on a beach blanket, and in the form of a half-dozen stuffed animals.

When visits are restricted and the patient's condition is best served by this, I often suggest tape recorded messages. With the use of a recorder and ear phones, patients, at their own discretion, can get audio reassurances from those they love.

If the patient is in a coma, I strongly recommend, with the physician's approval, an auditory and tactile program of stimulation. This approval may be hard to get, or it may be limited to certain types of comas. Some physicians may deny its effectiveness. But those who've worked in this field know better. Dr. Bernie Siegel, a surgeon from New Haven, Connecticut, has produced guided imagery and meditation tapes for comatose patients. He has learned that those in a coma, or under anesthesia, or asleep, still hear and, through instruction and practice, can alter the direction of their blood flow to assist with their own healing.

Stephen Levine, author of *Who Dies? An Investigation of Conscious Living and Conscious Dying*, recommends this approach: "If someone goes into a coma, stay with that person and talk with him. He is present. Indeed, coma is like being on the mezzanine. You are not yet on the second floor but you have a whole different perspective of the first floor. Talking with the person either aloud or silently through the heart seems to give a relative point, by which they can see that they are not who they imagined themselves to be, that consciousness is not limited to the body. Reading holy books and talking with someone who is in coma may be very useful to him . . . Music too may be of aid. Just be there."

If the patient has had a stroke, a head injury or brain damage of any kind, talk to the physician, speech therapist, physical therapist or others involved in the treatment about what you can do to help. If the patient is strong enough and willing, most medical personnel feel that early and continued stimulation brings a sense of well-being and is highly therapeutic when there's a potential for neurological recovery.

For those patients who have just experienced general anesthesia, the breathing exercises described in Chapter 3 will hasten the release of chemical residues still in the body and facilitate recovery and alertness. For those suffering from confusion, simple memory games that are pleasant and acceptable to the patient often help. Moreover, let every patient, *whether fully conscious or not*, know what is going on, what machines are being used and why, and what procedures and treatments are taking place. And as in other hospital situations, allow the patient as many choices as possible.

The most important element of all is your presence. For

those very seriously ill, focused attention through silence, meditation, prayer or work with the breath can often be the most healing treatment you can offer.

The main point is, don't be deterred. Dr. James Kelly, a Marin County, California, neurologist, says this: "I don't know if the positive effects of love and attention can be scientifically proven with my patients, but I know it *does* make a definite difference." Dr. Alan Teitelbaum, a San Francisco psychiatrist, says, "Patients usually can't remember the physical pain from an acute intensive care experience, but they can recall for years the emotional pain. Being with those they love can best prevent or lessen this type of pain."

THE MIRACLE OF LOVE AND ATTENTION

John's breathing was becoming more labored. As he inhaled, his long, slow intakes of air were rasping, erratic, a series of short, uncomfortable gasps and coughs, as if he were choking. As he exhaled, the rasping turned to a loud gurgling deep in his throat. He was sweating profusely.

Finding a wash cloth, Katherine wiped his brow. Then moving closer to his side she stroked him gently. "We're right here. You're not going to be alone."

Something about the way they looked on his cheek told Katherine they were tears. She pulled back to look at him. From his eyes, moisture was welling up and spilling down his face, forming wet spots on his gown. She put her hands to her face to see if they were not her tears. But she already knew they were his.

For a critically ill patient, the presence of a loved one can bring enormous benefits—from a release of emotion to a calming of fear and anxiety. A care partner arrangement

180

paves the way for close relatives and friends trained in appropriate behavior to play such a role, even in the innermost sanctums of intensive care.

Of course, it must be carefully planned and executed. Care partnering here must be done even more sensitively and consciously than that in any other part of the hospital. While the team can be formed by the same process—with one member developing the unit of three—the patient in critical care is usually much sicker and the chances for recovery more uncertain. There are many more nurses per patient, the rules are more restrictive, and the atmosphere is more charged with anxiety. Nonprofessionals must be given a higher level of training by their facilitator or the staff member on their team; and they must be more desensitized to what happens on such units. Most important, they must be more aware of the needs and requirements of the professional staff, who will need to be reassured that the nonprofessional presence will not impede vital medical procedures.

In this regard, the professional member of a care partner team or a staff person especially assigned to that function plays a vital role. That person becomes the educator and trainer for the family. He or she teaches them basic caregiving tasks that are medically and psychologically sound. And, far more delicate, he or she helps them negotiate with professional staff for a useful and respected role on the critical care team.

CHILDREN'S UNITS LEAD THE WAY

The children's units of many hospitals in this country have demonstrated that it can work. Dr. Louis Fine, Director of Psychiatric Liaison and Consultation Services in Denver's

Children's Hospital, attests to the value of including parents in the care of their critically ill children. "The provision of effective emotional care for children in a pediatric intensive care unit," he writes, "may help prevent a medical or surgical triumph from becoming a psychological disaster."

In a 1985 article on pediatric intensive care, Dr. Fine strongly recommends that parents become part of the critical care team. Through holding, feeding, soothing and reassuring their children, parents can become an essential element in their care program—listening to their concerns, changing their diapers and clothing, explaining the hospital to them and allaying their fears, just as would occur at home. "Parents may not know the medical/surgical nuances," writes Dr. Fine "(but) parents do know how to best soothe and parent their child."

The list of benefits that flow, not only to children, but to parents and hospital staff from Dr. Fine's approach almost exactly parallels the benefits of care partnering outlined in this book. For parents, it decreases the helplessness they feel; and by so doing, it reduces the competitive feelings they often develop toward staff. When their role and influence are acknowledged and valued, they are far more likely to cooperate with professionals whom they might otherwise suspect of usurping their function.

The University of California Medical Center in San Francisco has launched a "Care By Parent" program on its pediatric floors. The program has demonstrated that parents can be taught intensive nursing skills. For instance, they are taught how to care for colostomies, to administer chemotherapy, to do dialysis, to operate heart and breath monitors.

This interview extract, taken from an article published in the *San Francisco Examiner*, testifies to the success of the program. "'Most parents are terrified at first and overwhelmed,' says Lori Howell, a clinical nurse specialist for the program who serves in the facilitator's role. 'But our philosophy is that parents truly know the child best and that they can learn anything we can teach them as they room in with the child. Then in an emergency the parents can do the same thing we do—do CPR, give oxygen.' "

For children, the therapeutic effects are well documented. We now need to apply them more widely. Studies show that babies given standard physical care in institutions, but not special loving attention—not held, not sung to, not hugged—do indeed survive. But their development is slowed and their general well-being is not what it should be. Such long-standing findings should serve as ongoing proof that programs promoting love and attention in institutions must no longer be ignored. Holding, stroking and caring must no longer be limited to the young. They must be extended to all patients in all areas of the hospital, especially the critically ill.

If they aren't, we'll see more and more clinical observations noting "a failure to thrive." While first noticed in the studies of babies, such notations are being seen with increasing frequency in the medical charts of patients of all ages, especially the very old. And what makes them particularly poignant is that they're not a symptom of unsound medical practices. They're a symptom of unsound attitudes about the true nature of healing.

THE HEART OF HEALING

"What do you want?" Katherine asked her father. "You can come out of this coma, and if you decide on that, we'll see that you get the therapy you need. Or you can choose to die. You're the one who must decide."

183

"Hummm, humm," the doctor cleared his throat. He had come into the room so quietly that Katherine hadn't seen him. But he'd seen her; heard her, to be more exact. *"You still think he can hear, don't you?"* he asked, clearly intent on drawing a reaction from her.

Gathering her courage, she took him by the arm and walked him outside the door. *"Can you tell me 100% he can't hear?"* she asked.

"No," he answered slowly, *"no doctor could say that."*

Katherine put her hand on his shoulder and, turning him so they were face to face, she said, *"I know this is as hard for you as it is for us. None of us know precisely what to do. But this is what feels right to me,"* she explained. *"Since it can't hurt him, what's the harm? And maybe—just maybe—it might help."*

Sometimes we just don't know what to do. Some answers can never be clear-cut to anyone, not even doctors. But one sure way to *begin* making our way out of confusion is to start trusting our hearts. The heart requires no special training or education. It just knows the truth—or at least the truth as it applies to each of us. Often we forget that medicine is an art as well as a science. Intuition and instinctive "knowing" are crucial in the best medical care. This means that nonprofessionals can often "know" as much, if not more, than doctors about their own needs.

Norman Cousins respected his doctor's expertise, but he respected his own ideas as well. And even though his treatment plan, much of it based on the healing power of humor, had not been scientifically proven effective for patients in general, it proved to be exactly what *his* body needed. Now hospitals across the country are looking at the therapeutic importance of humor for all patients. Some believe that laughter has the same positive benefits for the body as jogging does. In effect, it's like an internal jogging session. The internal doctor in Cousins knew this all along.

184

Dr. LeBoyer proved what birthing mothers always knew. Babies should be delivered tenderly, with physical and psychological warmth, soft lights, quiet sounds and lots of loving contact.

When I first started working with the critically ill, I instinctively began to work with the breath. I had nothing to back my practice up. It just felt right. Now I've found that those more experienced in this work strongly recommend what my heart knew instinctively how to do.

Anya Foos-Graber in her book *Deathing: An Intelligent Alternative for the Final Moments of Life* gives specific instructions for breathing exercises that almost exactly parallel my experience. When Gregory Bateson was dying at the San Francisco Zen Center, the priest sent Zen students into his room and instructed them to breathe in unison with him as a way to deepen their empathy as they supported him in his release.

The principle of intuition is prized in the medicine of many cultures. The basics of Chinese acupressure and acupuncture, which have been effective treatments for over 3,000 years, were discovered through intuition. The ancient Chinese knew just where to apply pressure to remain healthy and to relieve tension and illness. These "inner teachings" were then passed down through the ages and ultimately codified. Similarly, the ancient teachings of East Indian yoga disciplines, still practiced today, came into being through meditation and intuition, not scientific experimentation.

Good psychotherapists and physicians—even though it is sometimes hard for the latter to admit it—rely as much on hunches and feelings as on training and technique. Dr. Jean Shinoda Bolen, a psychiatrist and author of *The Tao of Psychology: Synchronicity and the Self*, writes, "By our insistence that the scientific method is the only means by which anything can be known, doors of perception are closed, the wisdom of the East is denied us, and our own inner world becomes one-sided. East and West are two halves of a whole; they represent the two inner aspects of each individual man and woman. The psychological split needs healing through an inner union, allowing flow between left and right hemisphere, between scientific and spiritual, masculine and feminine, yin and yang."

When you are present with a person who is critically ill, listen to your feelings. Honor your intuition. Do anything that is important to you, as long as it does no harm. Healing is a sacred time. Don't hold back. Trust your heart.

It seemed almost certain now that John would not recover. But in the past weeks, those around him had learned to act from their hearts. And by so doing, they had grown, as individuals and as a family. They had touched base with their own hearts and then with the hearts of those around them.

Now Katherine wondered if they'd touched her father's heart. Had they reached the corners of his damaged muscles and tissues, penetrated the blockages that prevented his life's blood from doing its vital work? The scientist in her might argue and resist, but somewhere inside her, at a level deeper than the intellect, she knew they had.

There are no barriers to love, she told herself, no atherosclerosis of the emotional heart. Love was the miracle drug her family had to offer. It could go where pharmaceutical products could never penetrate—to the emotional and spiritual self. Everyone around her father had felt the effects of this potent love. Surely the patient, the person on whom they'd focused their attention, had felt it, too.

PART II: WHEN THE FAMILY MUST DECIDE

Starve John McGuire to death? Remove his feeding tube? It had never occurred to his family that this decision, like a deadly snake coiled in the grass, had been lying in wait for them all along. But John continued to live. His lungs continued to take in air and expel it. His heart continued to pump blood throughout his body. His brain stem was still alive. But what about his cortex—the place where, they were told, the man they loved would never reason or think again?

The option of removing his feeding tube was first broached to Katherine by Dr. Lloyd. It was then brought before Agnes, then Sarah and Teddy.

At first, paralysis set in. Removing the tube offered an end to their ordeal and a release for John. But denying their loved one food seemed somehow different from other "releases" from life. They shrank from the horror of playing God—from consciously opting for someone else's death.

But the issue was out in the open now, and they had to confront it.

The agony of those facing this question has been in the limelight since Karen Ann Quinlan's family, over 10 years ago, sought and won the legal right to remove their comatose daughter from her respirator.

Yet during that decade, as the number of families forced to make life-support decisions has steadily increased, we've learned little about how to ease them through it. Both the immediate pain and the long-term remorse imposed by the critical care experience have, if anything, grown more acute.

Many families simply acquiesce in the judgment of the doctor in charge. Others take matters into their own hands. In San Pablo, California, Edward Thomas Baker forced a nurse at gunpoint to remove his father from a respirator so he could die. In Milwaukee, nurse Thomas Engel, out of sympathy for a distraught daughter, disconnected the air supply of her rapidly sinking comatose father. In Los Angeles, Drs. Robert Nejdl and Neil Barber, with family approval, cut off the food supply of a near-brain-dead patient.

The consequences in each case were potentially tragic. Edward Baker and Drs. Nejdl and Barber were charged with murder. Wisconsin authorities threatened to suspend Thomas Engel's nursing license. But for our purposes here, the legal outcomes of these cases aren't the point. Regardless of how these cases were resolved in court, permanent emotional scars must have been inflicted on the people involved. Certainly since they hit the headlines, constant fear has become the companion of professionals everywhere. Indeed, for anyone who must live through—or work around—life-and-death decisions, the emotional trauma and beneath-the-surface fear can't help but be intense and ever present.

In fact, it can persist for a lifetime, often completely unrecognized by the doctors and nurses initially involved with families making these life-support decisions. We've discovered that many families, interviewed years later, are still suffering silent guilt, mutual recrimination and corrosive regret, because their decisions were made in haste, under pressure, and without adequate counsel and support. As for the health professionals—those who have pulled the plugs and removed the tubes—many of them are suffering, too, with little or no public, or even professional, awareness of the anguish *they've* endured.

WE'VE NOT SAT IDLY BY

In other areas, we've not sat idly by. During the past ten years we've developed all kinds of living wills and durable powers of attorney to cover health care decisions. Doctors and other health professionals have begun to regularly attend bioethical conferences. But do these measures really assure that those treating critical care cases and making life-support decisions will emerge from the experience fully informed and emotionally unscathed?

Hospital administrators, with the help of their attorneys, feel they've done everything possible to protect health workers. Health workers feel they've done everything possible to ease the burden of families. But ask any family who has recently contemplated removing a respirator or a feeding tube if they felt supported. Ask the doctor or nurse if he or she felt protected.

What's wrong? Why do we end up feeling so desperate? Why are we sometimes driven to extreme and destructive measures? Usually, it's because we've never fully understood our options. Feeling isolated and bewildered, we are easily frustrated, quick to conclude that the "legal remedies" purportedly designed to meet our needs are meaningless. For instance, when families try to enforce living wills, they often find these documents have no legal weight; or, when they are backed by legislation, the requirements for both living wills and the more popular durable powers of attorney contain more loopholes than protections.

Professionals, too, feel all alone, unable to fully rely on the goodwill of their patients and families or on the protection of their adminstrators or staff. They're simply not sure whether the family or the hospital will back them up in a court of law.

So we've become a society with the technology to defy death, but without an effective process for making the hard decisions which that entails. In fact, we've overlooked the *only* process which might be workable, the only one which we have any power to control. That is, some system like a care partnership which is fully in place ahead of time, designed to be automatically activated by hospital staff in moments of crisis, capable of supporting everyone across the board—the patient, the family and the professional staff handling the critical care issues.

CARE PARTNERING DURING
LIFE-SUPPORT DECISIONS

Care partnerships during these times should function somewhat differently from care partner arrangements elsewhere and at other times in the hospital. Here *every* patient and family making such critical decisions should be *guaranteed* a staff person to coordinate an education, counseling and support program especially for *that* family. This person would not be the attending physician nor the primary nurse nor any other staff involved in the direct medical care of the patient. He or she would act solely in the role of facilitator.

The role would be multifaceted. The facilitator would see that all parties involved have easy access to complete and current medical information, presented in a form that everyone could readily understand, about the illness in question. A second medical opinion would not have to be requested. It would be routinely offered. All available options (their benefits, drawbacks and possible consequences) would be explained. Information on who has the legal decision-making power (doctor, patient or family—and, if family, which member of it) would be reviewed, along with the ways to obtain that legal right, if needed. Appropriate and legal ways to record the decision would be gone over by all parties.

The facilitator would offer easy and immediate access to

190

a professional counselor, social worker, chaplain, minister or therapist. These would be individuals trained in listening to the feelings of patients, family and staff members, especially in cases where there is dissension within the family or among members of the staff.

Ideally, a group of experts would stand ready to advise. Many hospitals have bioethics committees made up of individuals representing different disciplines to assist and support staff dealing with situations like these. Teaching hospitals more and more are hiring bioethicists on their staffs to offer assistance. When a family wishes and needs extra help, a facilitator could ask for access to such a committee or call in an ethicist for help. But failing that, the facilitator would help families form their own panel of experts which they could work with individually or in a group.

Most important, once the decision was made, no matter what its content, the decisionmaker would receive continued support from the facilitator. Such continuity and support would be especially important in cases where an independent judgment did not coincide with what other staff or family members felt was "morally right," "economically feasible," "medically objective," or "traditional" in that community or hospital.

"NOT IN OUR HOSPITAL"

Administrators and their staffs, when presented with these possibilities, will respond with a litany of reasons why they are good in theory, but not practical or necessary—at least "not in our hospital." But to each objection, there's an answer.

Administrators will claim that they can't afford to hire new staff. But, in fact, the necessary staff is already in place. Chaplains, social workers, clinical nurse specialists in almost every hospital in this country are already trained and ready to serve. But these individuals usually have no authority to act without the referral of the physician or the request of the patient and family. Or they're authorized to offer only a part of the service—information but not counseling, counseling but no continued support.

Another reason given for not embracing this program is that "we already have it available in our hospital." All a patient or family member has to do is ask for it, professionals contend. This may be true. But by merely having it available, rather than integrating it into mainstream hospital procedures, they miss the point. Unless patients and families of all ages and circumstances are automatically informed of these services upon admission or at the time of crisis, it ends up being more form than substance. Unless a staff person routinely contacts every patient and family (without the necessity of a physician referral or without the family's self-initiated request) and works hand in hand with them to activate the process, it is rarely utilized in a full and meaningful way.

Recognition that there is a need for such automatic procedures is not new. Former President Jimmy Carter set up a President's Commission for the Study of Ethical Problems in Medicine and Biomedical and Behavioral Research, which first convened in January 1980. Its study extended through both the Carter and Reagan administrations. When its second and more highly recognized report was published in March 1983, this 554-page document *primarily called for hospitals to set up decision-making processes and procedures within their institutions to deal with the question of maintaining or foregoing life-sustaining treatment.*

Since that time much has taken place through bioethics

legislation and professional education. But little has been done in institutions to establish formalized decision-making procedures, at least in a mode that makes patients and families feel genuinely cared for and supported, and professionals feel understood and protected. Insurance statistics continue to prove that hospitals can reduce the number of claims against them if they would only begin to address these psychological needs. But for the most part hospitals have done very little in response.

Yet by ignoring these needs, they are imperiling everyone, including themselves. As we have seen, they have been subject to constant threats, sometimes at gunpoint, but more often in court. Moreover, these legal disputes are usually about much more than money. Contrary to popular belief, most malpractice suits are based on more than the desire to recover. The reasons behind them frequently have more to do with the human heart. They're more apt to be about feelings of powerlessness, pent-up anger, unresolved guilt and confusion, over how and why medical decisions were made and carried out.

For those who use drastic means to express their anguish, the consequences are obvious. They may lose their licenses or go to prison. For those who use more legal means, the fallout is more subtle. But, over time, it can be just as emotionally devastating.

And the tragedy is that far more often than not, none of this need have happened. The hospice experience provides the proof. Even though hospice patients are all terminally ill, and the family is almost always involved in the same type of critical decisions, when the patient dies, family members rarely feel this kind of anger towards hospice staff. The reason is the degree of patient and family education, counseling and support found within most hospice programs.

That fact should send a clear message to hospital and

nursing home administrators. At virtually no increase in cost or personnel, health care institutions could experience the same mutually agreed upon resolutions of critical care crises as do hospice organizations. And when patients die, families might be more interested in giving money to their hospitals in gratitude (as many now do to their hospice organizations) than in seeking to take money away from hospitals in courts of law.

The care partner approach, utilizing the concept of the POWER OF 3, offers hospitals a concrete way to introduce a comprehensive three-part program of education, counseling and support into critical care. It's time for hospitals and nursing homes to wake up. They simply can no longer afford to operate without some kind of formalized program like this.

But for patients and families acting alone, without an institutional structure, there are ways to help yourselves. First, find someone within the hospital to serve as your facilitator, and clearly outline your needs. Be sure to ask for all three parts of the program. Information is not enough. Insist on counseling and support as well. Then, begin by taking your time.

TAKING YOUR TIME

"I hope you won't act too fast," the aide said to Katherine as he lifted John up to sponge his back. "If you don't mind my saying so, Mrs. Hogan, it's better to take your time. I know. I was in a coma once. Stayed in it for two months before I came to."

Joseph, a powerful young black man, pressed a warm washcloth between John's shoulder blades, finding the muscles beneath the skin and massaging them in a steady, rotating movement. "The doctors

194

didn't think I'd make it. I remember one of them telling my folks, 'He's going to be a vegetable the rest of his life.' I heard him say that."

Joseph lifted his head, as if he were hearing the fateful words again. "I knew everything that was happening. I knew when it was raining from the sound on the building and all. I knew when the nurses were there, checking things. But I remember the doctors especially. They scared me . . . holding my hands, sticking pins in my face, treating me like a guinea pig or something."

Joseph's giant hands rubbed lotion into John's arms. Though he was the size of a football tackle, when he worked with a patient, he was like a mother with her child. "Do you miss your grandchildren?" he would ask John. "When you get well, I want to see you on that golf course, you hear?"

Joseph urged Katherine never to lose hope. "When I was out, I felt kind of cold and clammy, but my hearing was good—better than now. A person in a coma can think and feel. Don't ever forget that."

No matter how serious the condition, no matter how grim the diagnosis, most families wonder "what if?" What if my loved one is capable of recovering? What if we're acting prematurely? When large numbers of family members and/or professionals are involved, each individual can be at a different place along the continuum from indecision to decision, especially when the decision means withdrawing the patient from life-sustaining treatment.

Their hesitancy is understandable. We've all heard of that one person who beat the odds. Someone with the same kind of malignancy who survived the cancer. Someone six months into a coma who came out of it and lived. We've even heard of the woman with chronic pulmonary disease who insisted that if she were ever unconscious she should be removed from a respirator to die. But when that exact situation arose, and for some reason she was not removed, she got better and lived. On discharge she asked that her former life-support instructions be removed from her records.

No matter what our doctors say, we know there are no absolutes in life. There are always exceptions. We know the best the doctor can do is to offer us medical statistics. The evidence may be overwhelming against recovery; yet if the odds are one in a thousand, we wonder if our patient is that one.

My advice to those faced with any critical treatment decision is to ask for a timetable for coming to a conclusion, and within those parameters to take your time. You may find that the period you'll need to absorb and accept information emotionally is a lot longer than that required to process it intellectually. Using the care partner approach, with a facilitator assisting you, it should be possible for you to ask for and get all the time you need to satisfy yourself that the decision you make is the right one for you.

In the Appendix there is a set of twelve questions that you should ask yourself as you move through the decision-making process. They will help you resist rushing yourself—or being pushed by others—through this important transition from not knowing to knowing.

While certain family members may be able to satisfy themselves quickly about the right course to take, intense disagreement can still arise among the rest, between family and staff, or between staff and staff. Reaching consensus can be a formidable hurdle. For those groups still in contention, the best sequence of events is to first deal with the facts. Before you invest yourself deeply in a position, be sure you know who has the legal and final power to decide.

KNOWING WHO HAS THE FINAL SAY

There's a curious lack of knowledge in this country, even among medical professionals, about just who has the final legal authority to make treatment decisions in different sets of circumstances. This often leads to confusion and communication breakdowns, sometimes to tragedy. So it's time we got our decision-making rights straight.

In all legal jurisdictions in our country, the patient has the authority to make his or her own treatment decisions. The doctor may have to make quick judgments during the initial emergency, but any patient of sound mind has the ultimate say on whether that treatment should be continued, even if its discontinuation may lead to death.

When the patient is incapacitated, things get more complicated. Often misunderstandings arise over who exactly has the legal decision-making power. In most of these circumstances, the doctor has the right to make treatment decisions. That is, unless the patient is under eighteen. Or unless the state has passed a family consent act. Or unless another person has been designated as the patient's legal representative through a durable power of attorney arranged for earlier by the patient or through a conservatorship or guardianship awarded later by the courts. And with most legal actions, only *one* person is usually specified to exercise decision-making authority concerning health care.

Making critical treatment choices for other people is extremely difficult, and sometimes the person with the power does not want to assume the right. Often family members, when they have been granted this authority, prefer to hand it over to the doctors. Conversely, doctors, when they have legal authority, often want the family to direct them. In other instances, when one family member has been made legally responsible, he or she may opt to present the issue to other members of the family for a group decision.

There are many reasons why consensus is desirable. First, our society almost always views the family as having moral and social rights, even when members have no legal decision-making authority. Second, the medical profession at large is generally concerned about the risks of lawsuits. "This kind of situation must be dealt with very carefully," one East Coast internist has told me. "I insist that agreement be reached, or I persist with treatment . . . Otherwise I may be sued for malpractice." An internist at a bioethics conference in California put it this way: "I put the family in a room and tell them to duke it out until they decide."

Everyone is wise to expend time and energy on handling this process well. Not only is it important to know how every member of the family is feeling, the sensibility of the staff needs to be taken into account as well. The lawsuit cited earlier, charging the two Los Angeles doctors with murder, was not initiated by the family. A nurse unhappy about how the case was handled and the manner in which the decision was made was the person who brought the case to the attention of the District Attorney.

WHEN CONSENSUS COMES HARD

"Our family has never agreed on anything," Katherine said. "They tell us the family has to decide whether to take away Dad's feeding tube—as if, presto, we'll automatically see things the same way, just like that. Never mind that we can't agree on politics, religion, child rearing, or much of anything else. We're going to suddenly unite like magic and deal with this . . ."

198

She broke off, seemingly unable to go on. But then she continued. "Some of the family think he should be allowed to die. They feel he wouldn't want to live like this. So removing his feeding tube, they feel, would be a more loving act than keeping him alive."

She'd been talking steadily, ignoring the tears rolling down her cheeks and dripping onto her hands, clasped into tight fists in her lap.

"But that would be murder! When you remove a respirator, the patient still has a chance to breathe on his own. But the nutrition tube is a final act—more like holding a pillow over his mouth and nose until he suffocates and dies."

Katherine's sobs were now interrupted by hard dry choking sounds. She could hardly get her breath. Reverend Bingham offered her his handkerchief. She took it, wiped her face, then held on to it tightly.

"We're trying so hard to understand one another. But we've all gone through so much, tried so hard, and we're so tired."

Her head had slowly dropped. Now she was staring at the crumpled ball of wet linen clenched in her hand. But suddenly, as if the key issue had at last occurred to her, she looked up and blurted out her question.

"How can we get through this and still love each other as a family?

Throughout this book, I've talked about the value of facilitation in highly charged and subjective situations—moments of real or potential conflict when personal interests and most cherished values are at stake. The McGuires were in such a situation. Without this kind of help, most families have to tough it out on their own, making blind stabs at resolving their differences. More often than not, these families are like hostile armies in the night, lashing out with no clear idea of their own or their adversary's battle lines. Often they don't know exactly who their enemy is, much less how to sue for peace. So the wounds they inflict become doubly cruel. Inflicted arbitrarily and at random, they impose lifelong scars that need never have been.

With this family, Reverend Bingham saw the potential for just such a senseless battle. As its facilitator, he would ultimately need to have all parties interact with one another in the same room. But the situation he had in his office at that moment gave him an excellent opportunity to begin his work. He had a family member ready, indeed anxious, to speak honestly and unguardedly about her deep emotions.

He began by shifting the focus from the general to the personal. He encouraged Katherine to move from the family's feelings to her own. He invited her to reveal the contents of her heart—the "bad" as well as the "good."

"How do *you* feel about all this," he began simply. Then he sat back and listened.

What came out was her ambivalence—her fear that she could not go forward, her doubt that she'd be willing to retreat. Then there was her suspicion that she was behaving badly. Maybe she'd been a fool all along. Maybe everything she'd tried to do was simply wrong. Maybe by trying for a different kind of hospital experience for her father and everyone around him, she'd caused a lot of unnecessary trouble for nothing. But she'd felt so responsible for what was happening. It had seemed *she* was the one who had to make things come out right.

Reverend Bingham let her finish. By being nonjudgmental, he had let her know it was O.K. to feel the way she did. But then he went further, moving into the third step in the facilitation process. He validated her in her role as daughter and caregiver. He went over the good and positive things she had done for her father and family. "You know, the person who's been most blessed in all of this is your father. No matter what decision is made, John has had a daughter who's made his life beautiful right up to the end."

Without some release from this ambivalence—and in many cases, from intense criticism of others or of one's self—most people are unable to move toward resolution. Reverend Bingham clearly recognized that if the McGuire family was to come to consensus, each member would need to move through his or her own emotional process.

But for now the McGuires' struggle was not over.

HANDING OVER RESPONSIBILITY

Katherine didn't know what was happening. After all she had done day and night at the hospital and nursing home without tiring, now she felt helplessly and chronically fatigued.

Whereas before she'd felt like the Pacific Ocean—strong, forceful, pushing against all obstacles—now she felt like the creek on her family's farm, muddy and swollen after a fierce storm, but resigned to remaining within its own banks. All she wanted to do was lie on the couch, just as Agnes had done these past few weeks.

At the same time, Agnes was emerging as her old vigorous self. "Teddy, start the car," she said, putting on her lipstick and gathering up her purse. "You and I need to get to town. We've got to take care of John." Glancing at Katherine as she went out the door, she declared, "Nobody else seems up to it these days."

Robert Chernin Cantor, in his book *And a Time to Live*, describes the typical emotional responses of different personality types dealing with life-threatening illnesses. He distinguishes between the "reliant" and the "autonomous" personalities and their pros and cons. The reliant individual is willing to trust and rely on others to take responsibility. Anxiety is reduced by turning the responsibility over to a trusted authority person. However, feelings of helplessness and dependency can stem from this, as well as fears of abandonment.

When families face life-support decisions, I've observed that these individuals get by more easily at first. They turn over the hard choices to the attending doctor, the older sibling, the nurse, the minister, or almost anybody near at hand. Problems tend to develop only later, when these people suffer feelings of remorse.

"Why didn't I do things differently?"

"What would have happened if I'd spoken up?"

"How could I have made more of a difference?"

"If only . . . "

The autonomous personality behaves quite differently. Faced with a crisis, this person immediately goes into action—examines and re-examines all the options, seeks out and assesses information, tries to anticipate consequences. He or she moves vigorously to deal with the situation at hand. As a result, there is a strong sense of remaining in control, retaining personal independence and—as with the reliant person, but in different ways—keeping anxiety at bay.

But when life-support decisions must be made, autonomous people suffer greatly. By having assumed most or all of the responsibility earlier, they have made it extremely difficult to eventually "let go." When the time comes for acceptance and surrender, they continue to hang on.

And the hard truth that I've just recently come to recognize is that for family members to come through critical life-and-death decisions and emerge from the experience stronger, all parties must be willing to be *both* autonomous and reliant—at least to some degree and for a certain period of time.

All those with loved ones in the terminal stage will want, in the end, to feel they've done everything that was possible for them to do. But at some point in almost everyone's experience of this process, power and control must be relinquished.

ACTING FROM THE HEART

Reverend Bingham had talked to all of them during the past few weeks, separately and together. He'd focused particularly on those who had difficulty talking about feelings of helplessness, hopelessness, guilt and despair. He asked them to look particularly at those feelings generated by rage.

Because this family had a strong Christian heritage, and many of them still based their lives heavily on the scriptures, he chose to speak to them from a biblical frame of reference.

"Jesus expressed his humanness. In the garden of Gethsemane He was struck by waves of doubt and despair," he reminded them. "Why can't you allow yourself the same feelings?"

By posing his question in this way, the Reverend persuaded each of them to talk about the feeding tube, and at the same time, stay open to each other's points of view and emotional states. They discussed what each thought John would want—their personal perceptions of his beliefs, his personal values, what he'd wanted from life.

"We all know within us when to fight and when to surrender," Reverend Bingham told them. "We just have to listen inside for the answer. Listen while you pray or meditate. Pay attention to your dreams. That's where this kind of knowing sometimes comes to you. You can even ask John for a sign or a symbol. It might not come. Or it might come in a surprising or unexpected way. But whatever form

it takes, be ready to receive the answer. Something will let you know when it's time. Empty yourself of distractions and compulsions to control events, and just let it happen."

And one day it did happen. Maybe each of them, in his or her own way, had learned what each needed to learn. The way it happened was never clear. But in an unspoken but unmistakable way, they all came to know it at about the same time. They had made the decision.

The McGuires had someone guiding them who understood the subjective nature of such decisions. They were lucky. Some professionals don't understand. Many doctors believe that if life-support decisions are based on full and accurate information—if they've been arrived at after a reasoned weighing of the pros and cons—that should be sufficient. But it rarely is.

Granted, test results and statistics are important pieces of evidence. Our rational minds must be satisfied. In the back of this book, I cover the facts. I review the legal options. I give examples of living wills. I list states that have Natural Death Acts. I provide the names and phone numbers of agencies which support patients and families who have concerns about right-to-die decisions. I define "the codes" that hospitals use. I give information on organ transplants and funeral arrangements. But to the evidence of our rational mind must be added the evidence of our hearts. To be at peace with our final decision, we must come to terms with our whole person—our emotional as well as our logical selves. Only then can we make the move from knowing to accepting.

And those who can make their decision from the heart, no matter how difficult, will never resent the time or agony it took to get there. Such a decision is the only kind that truly sets us free. We are released, at last, to experience our grief without guilt or regret.

A TIME TO GRIEVE

But what about professionals? Do they experience grief? More important, do they experience release?

Some curious role changes occur in hospitals as the patient's prognosis shifts from the possibility to the probability of death. At the outset of the illness, particularly in cases when the family has been excluded from the hospital routine, when family members have just arrived from out-of-town, or when there are "autonomous" personalities within the family, some family members tend to feel personally responsible for all "caring" aspects of the patient's treatment. They feel they're there to buffer the patient from the professionals, those responsible for the more impersonal "curing" aspects. What's more, many professionals seem to accept that scenario. So while family members set about to bring comfort, affection and amusement to the patient, staff occupy themselves with numbers, reports and machinery.

But when the patient's prognosis worsens, these roles often become reversed. Family members once uninterested in the medical nuances become diligent students of the illness, challenging any procedure that seems suspect or ineffective and demanding input into every treatment decision. At that point, to fill the emotional vacuum created for the patient, many nurses tend to draw closer to the patient and to the role of emotional caregiver.

Still later, as the illness progresses, another shift takes place. Accepting the patient's death as inevitable, family members, needing space and time to work through their grief, tend to physically withdraw from the hospital altogether. As this occurs, the staff, in an effort to compensate, invest even more of themselves.

But while this sequence of events may be common—and indeed essential for the family—it is not necessarily good for everyone. At the time of death, staff have rarely taken the time to divest themselves of their emotions. Unlike the family, they have had no chance to work through their grief.

In these situations, the care partner program works to identify the needs of everyone involved, so that each, rather than responding unconsciously to the situation thrust upon him, can *choose* his behavior. Armed with this new awareness, the parties can select any role they want, including opting for the roles described above. But this time, they do it consciously. And they do it out in the open.

A family member can say, "I want more information." Another can declare, "I need to take time out for myself." A nurse can say to her superior, "I feel a need to spend more time with Mr. Johnson." When people are honest about how they feel, they can often sidestep misunderstandings, hurt feelings, anger and guilt. They can work through their feelings of hostility toward other people—as well as their self-recriminations.

Most important, a care partner arrangement allows for the lay person and the professional to have dual roles—as "carers" and "curers"—and to have them simultaneously. Moreover, at the end, both are accorded the time and opportunity to grieve. And, if they choose, to grieve together.

Admittedly, the care partner ideal is ambitious. But I'm convinced that it is doable. Acting in concert with the patient, as long as the patient is able, the POWER OF 3 *can* create new kinds of behaviors in our hospitals.

MAKING THE PROCESS YOUR OWN

Katherine was the first to speak. "I'll always remember sitting next to you in our old black Buick with the gray wool seat covers that tickled the back of my legs. You'd be driving me to school— seven miles along our bumpy road. First the hill and then the dip as we crossed the railroad tracks. You knew every curve in the road and everybody who lived along it. We'd wave and they'd wave back."

"Sometimes we'd just sit and say nothing. Sometimes we'd sing. You'd turn on the radio, and along with Tommy Dorsey and the Sentimentalists we'd harmonize. "Get your coat, don't forget your hat . . . "

The decision had been made. There were still tears, but there was no more paralysis. The pain, while still lurking just over the edge of consciousness, was being transmuted into something else. Something that felt right and good.

Despite their differences, Katherine and her family had sought and found ways of dealing with their grief. Throughout John's coma, because they were a family steeped in tradition, they had established rituals to move them through difficult times. Now they needed a way to tell John of their plans. That they would never forget him. But that they were emotionally ready to let him go.

So they conducted a type of service *with* John, focusing on him and his life and values. And since music and religion were important to him, religion and music became part of this ritual of letting him go.

Everyone got a chance to reminisce—to speak of the things they remembered most, the things about John that only the family would know. How, as an accountant who knew intimate financial affairs, he never charged anyone who was down on his luck. How, as a lover of golf, he'd sometimes play by himself, with the neighborhood dogs keeping him company around the course.

Funny, quirky things—things that couldn't be said about anyone in the world but John McGuire. That's what this ritual was about. A salute to a unique individual. A celebration of a never-to-be-repeated life. And a way for the family to transcend their pain.

Family members should choose how they want to participate in these decisions or whether they want to participate at all. And I'm suggesting not only participating in the decision, but if a life-support removal is chosen, in the removal as well. Although considered by some as unorthodox and by others as repugnant, every family should at least consider whether they would like to be involved when the respirator is disconnected or the feeding tube taken out. And if so, what way they would like to participate.

If you are one of those who wishes to be present at the removal, you must speak up. Unless you make your wishes known, you will probably be ushered out of the room. But you have every right to be present. And having made the decision to be there, you can make the most of the experience.

If you want to include poetry or music, make your selection. If you want flowers, bring them in. If you choose silence, ask that it be honored by staff. Do anything that is meaningful to you and to those you love. By the same token, if you choose to remain in the waiting room or at home, find some way to use that time in a way that reflects your values and the depth of your feelings.

By so doing, you will have grasped a truth that health professionals still struggle to learn—that the answer to the life-support dilemma can never be solved by arriving at the "right decision." The "right decision" changes with social mores, as sand patterns change with time. The "answer" can only be found in the "right process," in a method that allows patients—or when that's not possible, family members—to question and challenge, then create their own ways of moving toward resolution.

A BETTER WAY

The family had now circled John's bed.

"Though I speak with the tongues of men and angels, and have not love," Reverend Bingham began, "I am become as sounding brass, or a tinkling cymbal . . . "

Katherine, standing head bowed, saw them all in her mind—the medical and hospital staff, the nursing home staff, its residents, the sitters. Their love had been palpable these past few weeks, and she could feel it now, suffusing John and his family in its warm, supportive glow.

"John, honey," Agnes said. "We've come to say goodbye. You can leave us now. We're strong enough now to let you go. And we've all agreed." As Agnes told her husband of the family's decision to no longer fight his death, Katherine mused over these last few weeks. So many things were becoming clear to her. Death had never been their enemy, she now realized. Dying had been—unconscious dying. Dying while those around remained unconscious, unaware. Their triumph had been that, through John's coma, they had changed, become aware. And in their efforts to raise John's consciousness, they had raised their own.

The minister prayed. "Give us faith to see beyond touch and sight, some vision of Your kingdom. When vision fails, give us trust of Your love which never fails."

Each of them hugged John. Then they turned and hugged one another. Finally they left together to complete their final task.

At the nurses' station they presented the head nurse with a

piece of paper with some writing on it. "This is what we want,"
Agnes told her. "We want it put in John's chart."

Realizing the importance of the moment, the nurse read the
instructions out loud.

January 11, 1983

TO BE PLACED IN THE MEDICAL CHART OF JOHN ARTHUR McGUIRE:

We, the family of John Arthur McGuire, would like all doc-
tors, nurses, anyone associated with John McGuire's care to
know it is our request that you do NOT aggressively treat any
medical complications. This would mean no antibiotics for fe-
ver, infections or pneumonia. This would mean no supplemen-
tal oxygen.

We would, however, expect you to continue giving him the
basic level of nutrition and hydration. Keep him as comfortable
as possible and continue to give him emotional as well as physi-
cal support.

Thank you for your care. Thank you for your concern.

Signed,

Agnes Matthews McGuire
Katherine Ann Hogan
Theodore Morgan McGuire
Sarah Alice McGuire

So the McGuires, following their own sometimes painful
process, had emerged as a family intact. Despite often bitter
dissension among themselves, and sometimes between them
and hospital staff, they had found their way.

But how much better it would have been if they had
found what they needed *because of* "the system" rather than *in
spite of* it. How much better if a care partner program had
been in place, ready to be activated that very first night, when

210

Katherine pushed through the hospital's heavy glass doors with fear and apprehension in her heart.

It can happen. It must happen for every person involved in critical care decisions. The secret to resolution and eventual release for patients and family members lies in empowering them—making them full members of the health care team—and in recognizing that the critical care experience must largely be determined by them. Until the people whose lives are most affected can feel good about their process—asking every question they want to ask, consulting with every specialist they need to see, working through their crisis on their own terms and feeling supported in their struggle—they will never feel at peace with its outcome.

And neither will the professionals with whom they work.

THE SILENT SUFFERERS

When I've interviewed professionals about their response to the critical care experience, I've found they've had little opportunity to integrate their feelings. When I ask questions about life supports, I get mixed responses—from doctors who say they feel no emotional repercussions after removing tubes to nurses who worry about how they'll be dealt with on "judgment day."

"It's simple," one internist replied when asked what it's like to remove someone from a respirator. "You take a syringe and deflate the pressure gauge around the tube, and then pull out the tube. It takes about five to ten seconds."

He denied that the experience had any emotional content. "It's nothing," he assured me. "I'd take my own father off one and never bat an eye."

But when the same question was asked of a nurse in the

211

hospital where this doctor worked, she gave a more revealing answer. "It's something I worry about a lot, that most nurses worry about, although we rarely discuss it." About herself, she said, "I only hope God knows that I do my best, and that I wouldn't deliberately do anything wrong."

About the doctor quoted above, she said, "Doctors say there's no problem for them to remove life supports, but that's because *they* don't do it. They have us do it."

When I probed deeper into the doctor's statement, she said, "Look, I've been working in this hospital going on twelve years, and I've only heard of one doctor who's ever carried out his own life-support order. They have as hard a time as we do, but they just don't admit it."

We must look at better ways for professionals to deal with their feelings on these issues—both those expressed and those unexpressed; both those acknowledged and those denied.

Three days later John McGuire died of a high fever and an acute infection.

The following day, without an appointment—but with the blessings of the front office—Katherine walked into Dr. Lloyd's consulting room. He stood near his desk. His familiar white coated back, slightly rounded through the shoulders, was turned to her.

Intently studying a file folder he had in his hands, he saw Katherine from the corner of his eye and turned in surprise, startled out of deep concentration.

Confronted with the same quizzical look, the same bifocals adjusted down on his nose, Katherine felt the old dread in her stomach. But she plunged on, "The family has something important to say to you." The frown line deepened between his eyes.

"Thank you," she said, looking straight at him. "Thank you for all you've done."

Gathering himself together, he motioned her to sit down and settled himself behind his desk. "I'm sorry for all the trouble I caused you," she said. "I realize I must have been really difficult for you at times. If I had to do it over, there are things I'd do differently. But in the really important things, I know I'd have to do what I did all over again."

He looked down at his hand still holding the file folder, one finger inserted in the place where he'd left off. "I wouldn't say you were difficult," he said stiffly, stretching to be precise, to define his position exactly. "I thought your idea of being able to communicate with your father was unrealistic. I still do. And from the point of view of the hospital, it was highly irregular for you to spend the night in the Coronary Care Unit. But you arranged to do it in such an unobtrusive way . . . " His words trailed off, as if he were lost in memory, reconstructing his experience of that time. "And it seemed to mean so much to you . . . "

He was silent for a moment. The day outside was overcast, and the light in his office was subdued, placing one side of his face in shadow. But the other side stood out, its details deeply etched by the light of his reading lamp. Katherine thought she saw a film of tears glistening behind the protective shell of his glasses.

"You know," he said, "it's hard to see a man who's been your patient for years—someone who's become a friend . . ." He paused to control his voice, then began again. "It's so frustrating. Here was a man who'd gone through by-pass surgery and seemed to be doing so well . . . "

Taking out a large white handkerchief, passing it over his eyes, he sat in silence. After a moment Katherine spoke, "I've learned so much from this experience. Do you think you have?"

He leaned back in his chair and looked beyond her, "One of the Greeks said, 'I'm part of all I've met.' I tend to believe that."

Then, not really speaking to her but more to himself, he mused, "The funny thing is, no one's asked me before how I felt about these things . . . No one's ever asked."

213

Chapter 8

THE CALL FOR REVOLUTION

The sceptical reaction I sometimes get when I suggest that individuals are capable of making significant changes in large institutions is understandable. My listeners are normally people outside hospital and nursing home circles who imagine they have little power within institutional walls. But curiously enough, when I've approached health professionals about how they can effect change in their own environments, I get an amazingly similar response. I call it the "yes, but" reaction.

"Yes, I like what you're saying, but you're really only writing to a small minority of patients and family members, maybe less than 1%."

"Yes, I agree, but your approach takes too much staff time, more staff than we have in our small hospital."

"Yes, this might have worked before Medicare cut-backs, but not now. Patients are in and out too fast."

"Yes, but ... but ... but ... "

These are well-meaning people, forward looking and

open to change. But they see themselves as realists, careful not to reach for the impossible.

So let me speak in "realistic" terms. It's too late for rationalizations. A reform movement is already underway—and it's happening in that most powerful of all places, at the grass-roots. Lay people are demanding that patients and family members be treated with respect. They are calling out for hospitals and nursing homes that listen and respond. And they're prepared to fight to get them.

Some health professionals are beginning to listen. Some are questioning the way they're forced to do business. And they're putting their jobs on the line to speak out. What's more, hospital administrators are listening, too. They know that unless there are immediate changes for the better, their institutions may soon be out of business.

Just look at the evidence of the market place. What better way to confirm what's happening than to watch those spotters of trends, the market researchers. The same marketing minds that tell Proctor and Gamble what housewives want in detergents are telling hospital administrators what patients want in health care.

And what they're saying is that hospitals must be more hospitable. On that point, I agree. But that's where our agreement ends. Their version of hospitality is, in many ways, worse than what it replaces—promising more, but often delivering less, and charging double for the pretense.

Later in this chapter, there'll be more on "hospitality hospitals" and why most fall short of the real thing. But for now, let me suggest what I believe *is* the real thing.

The real thing springs from the heart. And it is usually, if not always, set in motion by one person. It can be initiated by extraordinary individuals with great wealth and influence,

216

with exceptional talent, with high professional standing. Or it can be carried out by ordinary people like most of us.

But most of us want someone else to make the change. It's so much easier to call for change than to *be* the change. Most people feel they don't have sufficient power or leverage in institutions to influence them, even though some are working inside them and some are paying their bills. But once these individuals begin testing their autonomy and power, they find they have more of both than they first realized.

So we'll look at stories of people who have made significant changes in hospital care. Initially, they all had their doubts. But they accomplished what they did because their power came from their ability to care. And because they cared, they managed to transcend the rationalizations, the "good reasons" for not acting, and followed their hearts.

THE LAY PERSON AS ACTIVIST

One extraordinary person was Planetree's founder. In the course of one year, Angelica Thieriot found herself virtually living in hospitals, first as a patient with a mysterious and life-threatening virus, then as a mother with a son desperately ill with osteomyelitis, then as a daughter-in-law whose husband's father was dying of cancer. And, to her shock and horror, all three experiences turned out to be "nightmares." Apart from the gravity of the illnesses involved, the hospital experience itself was dehumanizing and worked against rather than for healing.

The experience left Angie Thieriot with a firm resolve—to make things better. She determined to create a new kind of hospital, where patients and families would be treated with dignity and respect.

"Many of the most important moments of people's lives are spent in hospitals," she reasoned. "Yet, for the most part, they're the coldest and ugliest places on earth. Why can't a hospital feel like a spa? Not just for the rich, but for everyone. Why can't it feel good to walk into one? I just don't believe it can't be done."

Combating the "Yes, Buts"

The first step was taken in 1981 with the establishment of the Planetree Health Resource Center in San Francisco, a place mentioned earlier in this book, where lay people could go for health information. It was a beginning. But Angie, whose philanthropic interests had already been extensive, wanted more than that. She wanted across-the-board changes, a new humanistic approach to health care. It took her seven years to get it.

Several foundations were interested in her ideas, but they remained noncommittal. She would have to secure a space, they said, before she could come back to them. But finding a host hospital wasn't easy. Most hospital administrators replied politely that no extra space was available. Some had space, but were unable to comprehend her vision, and so found other excuses to say "no." Two hospitals offered specialty units—one in oncology and one in pediatrics.

But Angie held out for the "impossible." She insisted that this opportunity be available to anybody who needed hospital services. She argued for a straight medical/surgical ward; and she wanted it placed in a well-established teaching hospital. So she prodded and pushed until the administrator of Pacific Presbyterian Medical Center in San Francisco said "yes."

After the ideas and planning came the implementation.

Architectural blueprints were drawn and redrawn. Items most contractors never think to question, the Planetree architect questioned. "Why are the oxygen and suctions panels permanently fixed on the side of the wall, so patients have to be turned *away* from the bay view?" she asked. "And why don't the windows open for fresh air?"

Endless meetings were held with fire marshals, building inspectors, state licensing representatives, anybody who had some say in how health care facilities should be built. "You can't have a refrigerator for patient use on the floor," they ruled.

"Why not?" Angie countered. "There're refrigerators for every other use—for blood samples, for tissue specimens, for staff food. Why not for patient food?"

The easiest of tasks often created the most uproar. Angie wanted a shelf positioned along the wall of every room, where patients could easily place pictures and other personal items brought from home. "They'll be too hard to clean," the housekeeping department objected. "They'll get knocked down and create safety hazards," the hospital engineers cautioned. Angie persisted.

In the end, she got her refrigerator. She got her shelves. She got an agreement from administration to experiment with some unprecedented patient care policies. And on June 3, 1985, she got the Planetree Model Hospital Unit.

The Shift to "Yes, And"

That unit is now five years old, but its standards are as high as they were at the outset. Only certain doctors can admit their patients to Planetree; and only certain nurses are selected to work there. They must have demonstrated a strong commitment to the philosophy of patient education. They must believe in patient participation and family involvement in the treatment plan. And they must be able to tolerate the frustration and uncertainty that accompany experimentation.

"Planetree has something to offer everyone," says one patient. "Education for the patients who want education and gentleness and comfort for the patients who just want to be taken care of. And music and movies and pretty rooms. If you have to be sick, this is the place to be."

What's more, hospitals and professionals around the country are taking note. On August 7, 1987, at the annual meeting of the Association of Humanistic Psychology, the Planetree Model Hospital Unit was awarded the Gertrude S. Enelow Award for outstanding accomplishments in humanizing hospital care. And on October 22, 1987, Ms. Theiriot was presented with the Easter Seal Society award for outstanding public service in the field of health care.

Angelica Thieriot was after complete reform when she pioneered Planetree. She worked from the theory that "one way to judge a society is how well it takes care of its sick and fallen members." Refusing to listen to the "yes, buts," she insisted on a philosophy which called for "yes, and."

THE PROFESSIONAL AS CATALYST

Here's the story of a physician who changed the entire climate of a cancer research unit in a large university hospital. Dr. Samuel Klagsbrun, a psychiatrist, later wrote about his experience in the *American Journal of Psychiatry*.

The patients on this ward were there for research purposes. If their cancer went into remission, they were immediately discharged for outpatient services. In other words, those remaining were the difficult cases, often referred to by staff as "the walking dead." But like most hospital units, the staff didn't talk openly about their feelings, especially regarding those who were dying or (in the minds of the staff) already dead. Instead, they suppressed their dismissive and angry feelings. Then they suffered silent guilt for having had them at all.

The patients were not a happy lot, either. Besides the pain and fear they suffered from their illness, they complained about being guinea pigs and talked to anyone who would listen about the "uncaring doctors" and "unavailable nurses."

Dr. Klagsbrun felt the patients' morale and behavior would improve if they could see themselves as functioning and productive members of society. As the psychiatric consultant to the unit, he decided to create what he called an "antiregressive atmosphere." He determined to address staff and patients as functioning adults and encourage them to reach within themselves, examine their feelings and discover their autonomy and power.

He began with the nurses. He knew that in order to draw from them an unguarded expression of their feelings, he needed to begin these sessions within their level of comfort. He started simply, soliciting and answering questions about prescribed medications and types of cancer treatments.

But as Dr. Klagsbrun gained the nurses' trust and confidence, they started opening up about personal feelings. They began realizing it was all right to express negative attitudes, to air grievances and to propose solutions to them. In short, an environment had been created in which problems could be safely explored; and, even more important, in which the nurses themselves were urged to take responsibility for solving them.

When nurses began to see themselves as no longer victims

221

of circumstances beyond their control—as not permanently operating under the thumbs of doctors, but as agents of change—things began to happen. As they found their power, they encouraged the patients to find theirs. More activities were encouraged inside the ward. Passes out of the ward were issued, when appropriate. Most important of all, patients were taught how to care for themselves.

Walking through the ward on any day, you could begin to see patients making their own beds and fetching their own ice and water. That's not to say there weren't mixed reactions among them—some felt challenged, others felt even more abandoned and rejected by staff. But the patients themselves handled these problems. The active among them began to take care of the less active—making their beds, bringing them their water. They began taking on desk jobs, answering phones and typing forms. The more experienced ones assumed responsibility for orienting new patients.

As patients began to work together, they also began to eat together, then to play together. Card games and jigsaw puzzles began appearing everywhere. Their will to live had clearly increased. It was as if they were saying, "Don't count us out. We're not dead yet."

The other doctors on the ward took notice. As they became more interested in what was happening, they spent more time with the patients. They grew less distant with the nurses. Instead of reacting critically to the nurses' education program, they became intrigued by it. And with time, the nursing turnover rate not only decreased, but new nurses requested to work in this hospital and on this ward.

What had happened, then, was a chain reaction. Starting with an improvement in the quality of the nurses' work experience, the reaction had spread from one group to another, until the entire culture of the ward had been transformed. The job of its catalyst, Dr. Klagsbrun, was over. He had little left to do but watch its benefits spread.

ORDINARY PEOPLE AS TREND SETTERS

What can we learn from the Thieriot and Klagsbrun stories? Surely not just that these gifted and well-placed individuals happened to be successful in two isolated situations. Surely their experiences say something about what any ordinary person can do to change his or her hospital experience— and by so doing, become part of the cumulative effort fueling the movement toward hospital reform.

Take the example of the ordinary women of the 1970s who, acting one by one, pushed hospitals into childbirth reforms. Only twenty years ago or less, women giving birth in hospitals could expect standard OB procedures—enemas, pubic shaves, large doses of medication and anesthesia. The mother labored and gave birth without support from her loved ones. Her baby was taken from her at birth. While in the hospital, she was allowed to see her newborn only a few minutes a day, and never to take over the basic parenting tasks which she had waited so long to perform.

Obstetricians were not the ones to cry out for change. OB nurses led no movements toward reform. Confronted with signs of rebellion, health professionals, for the most part, dug in their heels. It was the pregnant women of America who demanded childbirth education, "birthing rooms," family involvement in the birthing process, and "rooming-in" for their babies.

Predictably their demands met with standard responses.

"Childbirth education takes too much time."

"Women are in and out of the hospital too fast these days."

"Most women don't want to know these things."

"An alternative birth center? Nonsense! "

"The father in the operating room? Outrageous!"

"The family helping with the delivery? Out of the question! This is a hospital, not a family reunion."

But women persisted. They had no organized group to back them. For the most part, they didn't think to organize themselves. Each woman knew what she wanted for herself and her family, and each woman, acting as an individual, pushed for change.

They succeeded beyond all expectations. Today, obstetricians wouldn't dream of returning to the days of uninformed patients, of anxious mothers paralyzed by fear and drugs. OB nurses wouldn't think of acting without family involvement. Both insist that fathers have an important role to play. Both insist on the psychological necessity of early infant bonding with loved ones.

And they're not alone. Hospital administrators insist on modern birthing rooms, complete with double beds and patterned wallpaper. In fact, their conversion provides the most convincing proof of all that the childbirth movement has been good for everyone—babies, mothers, families, health professionals *and* hospitals.

THE LAY-PROFESSIONAL PARTNERSHIP

As we have seen, it is almost always an individual— sometimes a professional, but usually a lay person—who speaks out first for a more sensitive, personalized environment for hospital patients. But once that happens, the impetus it provides can lead to a partnership, a collaboration, and ultimately a movement. So it was with the hospice movement. The relationship between David Tasma and Dr. Cicely Saunders, the patient/inspirator and the physician/founder of London's St. Christopher's Hospice, was just such a partnership. And, in time, Saunders took Tasma's vision and made it a reality.

"It was through David's eyes that I was given the vision of this hospice . . ." Dr. Saunders was quoted as saying in Sandol Stoddard's book *The Hospice Movement.* "As he was dying in a busy surgical ward, we talked for many hours of what his real needs were—not simply for medical care as such, but for someone to care for him as a person, to stand by and honor him for what he was—and it was he, a refugee from the Warsaw ghetto, who left the first 500 pounds for St. Christopher's."

Dr. Saunders recalled Tasma's last request. "'I want what is in your mind and what is in your heart,' he told me. I saw then that what was needed was a place that was both a hospital and a home; and he said, 'I want to be a window in your home.' We have many windows here."

From that small beginning came St. Christopher's Hospice, which has become the model and inspiration for the development of more than 1500 hospice organizations in the United States over the last decade.

A hospice, as defined by Dr. Saunders, is a place where patients can receive protection, refreshment, fellowship and cherishing as an integral part of their medical care. But in order for this to happen, she feels, such a center needs to be located *outside* the typical hospital setting.

Many respected authorities, both inside and outside the medical field, have agreed with her. Dr. Elisabeth Kübler-Ross strongly advises her patients to die at home rather than subject themselves to the degradation of hospital environments. Most hospice organizations in this country have centered their activities around home care alternatives rather than institutional care. Agencies funded under the Older Americans Act are mandated to provide services that avoid or delay institutionalization of older people. Even doctors are setting up their own surgery and urgent care centers, so they will no longer have to work in hospital settings. People in general, no matter what their age or degree of illness, when given a choice, prefer to work or be cared for anywhere but in large, complex health facilities. When Norman Cousins was a patient, he moved himself into a hotel for his convalescence. He summed up his feelings this way: "A hospital is no place for a person who is seriously ill."

HOSPITALS: NO PLACE TO BE SICK?

But let's not deceive ourselves. Institutions are and will continue to be an essential part of our health care system. Given that fact, we must demand that hospitals and nursing homes learn how to care. We can support home services, even surgery centers, and at the same time seek radical changes *within* institutional walls. But in order for these changes to have permanent impact, we must first have fundamental reform.

The need for reform can hardly be questioned. Health care institutions, as they now operate, often lead not to recovery, but to death. If that seems a harsh judgment, consider this. By causing social, emotional and spiritual pain, they can eventually cause social, emotional and spiritual death. That, in turn, can lead to physical death, sometimes prematurely.

That hospitals routinely inflict social, emotional and spiritual pain has been well documented by such respected authorities as Dr. Richard Kalish, Professor of Behavioral Sciences at the Graduate Theological Union in Berkeley, and Dr. Robert Woodson, Director of the Santa Barbara Pain Clinic. Dr. Kalish warns families that social death can happen any time a seriously ill person enters a hospital or convalescent home.

Consider the difference between the traditional hospital and a healing environment such as I'm proposing. In my model, helping the patient find meaning and purpose in illness (indeed in the full sweep of the life experience) is regarded as fundamental to the healing process, whether the outcome is expected to be recovery or death. But in the typical hospital environment, a patient's need to participate in some personally meaningful experience or ritual is often blocked by the isolating nature of the institution and by the indiscriminate use of sedatives and drugs. Except in those few situations where a chaplain is on staff, spiritual pain is never acknowledged, much less addressed by most health professionals.

In short, whether they intend it or not, hospitals, by the very manner in which they operate, are not unlike prisons. They dehumanize their patients—removing their clothes, taking away their possessions, limiting their opportunities to be with loved ones, restricting their expressions of personal feelings and their opportunities for learning and growth.

Dr. M. Scott Peck, a psychiatrist and author of *People of the Lie: The Hope for Healing Human Evil*, goes even further. In his view, institutions have the potential for doing "evil." While we may shrink from his choice of language, Dr. Peck's choice is deliberate. He assigns a precise meaning to the word "evil," and he employs it with a distinct purpose. Evil, according to Dr. Peck, is anything which kills the spirit of another person.

"We are living in the Age of the Institution," he writes. "A century ago the majority of Americans were self-employed. Today all but a small minority devote their working lives to larger and larger organizations . . . As they become larger and larger, (these) institutions become absolutely faceless. Soulless."

What's worse, in institutions where staff members are under chronic stress, a kind of "psychic numbing" can take place, even on the part of those assigned to healing roles. Dr. Peck speaks of this: "When we are insensitive to our own suffering, we tend to become insensitive to the suffering of others." Hence, he cautions us to watch out for institutional settings where obedience is valued more than autonomy. He alerts us to specializations which allow individuals to pass the "moral buck," to environments where the indignities workers suffer prompt them to pass on those indignities to others. Technology, which can help people get well, can also lead to emotional distancing, he concludes, and that can lead to "evil" as he defines it. Thus, the task before us, as he sees it, is to "metaphorically exorcise our institutions."

This implies a kind of self-purification process within our facilities. Yet institutions are rarely eager to change themselves. Rarely is a group willing to conduct the painful self-examination needed for change. So it is up to the individual to take direct responsibility for that change. "As a single vote may be crucial in an election," Dr. Peck writes, "so the whole course of human history may depend on a change of heart in one solitary and even humble individual."

MOVING FROM THE DATA TO THE DOING

We haven't a moment to lose. "Our ability to move our (hospitals) toward superior customer responsiveness," warns Richard Stier of the *Healthcare Forum*, "will largely determine our ability to survive during the next four years—a period that innovation expert Lee Kaiser has called the 'shakedown period' (for hospitals)." Tom Peters, co-author of *In Search of Excellence* and *A Passion for Excellence*, puts it in a somewhat different way, but the message is the same. "Superior responsiveness to customers," he writes, "results in superior financial performance."

And there are data to back this up. The Strategic Planning Institute conducted a 20-year study of two groups of manufacturing and service businesses—those that customers rated low in quality of service and those they rated high. The findings clearly bear out the hypothesis that superior responsiveness to customers does result in superior financial performance.

The management at Porter Memorial Hospital in Denver, Colorado, conducted 17 focus group interviews in 1984, 1985 and 1986. The groups were composed of former patients, families of former patients, potential patients, and patients of competing hospitals. Asked what they most wanted in hospitals, the responses of all groups were similar: "More one-on-one attention." The thread running throughout was this: Patients want understanding, support, even love, while in a hospital.

Richard Stier, in his 1987 article "The Economics of Patient Satisfaction," described a follow-up to the Denver focus groups. Because of the limited sample size and qualitative nature of the Denver data, the Ireland Corporation was hired to conduct a more quantitative study. Using standard research methods, the Ireland group conducted a telephone survey of

229

1,450 patients and potential patients living in the Denver area during the same three years as the Porter Memorial Hospital study.

The top two hospital selection criteria cited by 98.8% of the respondents during each of the three years were: "Keeps patients informed about their condition," and "Is attentive to the needs of patients and their families." Interestingly enough, other criteria, such as, "Provides good nursing care," "Offers the latest medical equipment," "Has a good reputation," and even "Has reasonable prices," did not score nearly as high as the top two cited above.

Hospital administrators are well aware of their financial bottom line. They're ready to try new approaches to bring patients into their hospitals. They are searching for ways to move from the data to the doing; but most simply don't know how.

HOSPITALITY HOSPITALS: ARE THEY FOR REAL?

In an effort to attract more patients and/or to cut costs, many hospitals are beginning to package and advertise special patient services. Terms such as "hospitality hospitals" and "cooperative care institutions" are cropping up across the country.

One hospital brochure poses a series of inviting questions: "Do you want a guest bed in your private room for your spouse or friend? Do you want a teddy bear and chicken soup? Basket of flowers? Gourmet picnic basket for two? Facial? Massage? Movies? Secretary? Phone dictation? Our hospital brings you services you normally enjoy at home or at the office—or in restaurants and beauty shops."

Some of these services are included in overall hospital

fees; but most come with an additional price tag, ranging from $15 for a manicure to $70-$225 per day for a luxury suite. These VIP quarters often feature antiques, fine rugs, silver-handled doors and, at one hospital, 19th-century oak fireplaces. At a hospital in Bethesda, Maryland, patients get breakfast—and a rose—on a silver tray. In the evening, they're served an exotic dinner from a famous Washington, D.C., restaurant.

My advice to anyone intrigued by these blandishments is: BEWARE! Hospitals are desperate. Undercut by dwindling government support, changes in insurance policies and demands for less expensive outpatient services, many facilities are either closing their doors or looking for more aggressive marketing strategies. One of these strategies is to hire marketing consultants with business backgrounds and hotel executives with guest relations training, who promise to help hospitals gain substantial profits, some at the patients' expense. And in so doing, these outsiders are recommending a shrewd new approach—in essence, a clever imitation of patient-centered health care.

"We're finding that people don't look at the diplomas on the wall," reports Robert Erra of the Santa Barbara Medical Foundation in a 1985 article in *Newsweek*. "Instead they want to know if the hospital is clean, if it has friendly receptionists, if the doctors are warm and caring."

So hotel management training has found its way into health care institutions, bringing with it gourmet menus, special crystal and china, coordinated bed linen, patient entertainment, home-style conveniences and programmed courtesies. In packaged seminars, costing anywhere from $2,000 to $20,000, Marriott and other corporations are giving hospital staff special training in patient interaction—the art of conversation, of reading body language, of handling the *customer.* Staff are carefully coached in the niceties of this system: "Make eye contact. Introduce yourself. Call people by name. Explain what you're doing."

Some hospitals are doing well using the new approach, despite occasional resistance from staff. The program at Albert Einstein Medical Center in Philadelphia did not begin without internal opposition. "There was some resentment," recalls psychologist Stephen Stelzer. "The hospital was telling people to be friendly, and most people thought they were doing it already." But the patients noticed a difference. They began telling their friends about it, and the hospital census started to increase. The bottom line had spoken loud and clear. The program was deemed a success.

Moreover, those hospitals that have been successful in repackaging their image have joined Marriott in merchandising their new expertise. Einstein has begun to sell its program to at least four other hospitals, projecting profits in the range of $150,000.

The hotel industry isn't alone in getting into the "health business." Video companies are competing to serve the "bored patient" and the "working doctor." Each offers patient entertainment tapes similar to those shown on airplanes. These can be anything from comedy shows to health education. One, a hospital comedy show, is named "In Stitches." The price tag is steep. For example, American Network charges $5 a month per bed, plus a flat monthly fee of $1,200 per hospital. Such costs are passed on to the doctors and patients who use the services.

The emerging pattern is often one of commercialism run rampant. And the danger is that it's hard to really know that from the outer package. Most of these programs are developed with Madison Avenue slickness. They may sound good—in fact, exactly like what has been proposed in this book. But there's a crucial difference. Most are in the business of manipulating patients rather than serving them. Even though some represent a step in the right direction, *control remains with the institution and is rarely if ever shared with the patient.*

Under these circumstances, promises are often made without commitment or substance. While reading a full page ad about new hospital services in a local hospital recently, I was intrigued by an announcement about a patient education service, said to be a new feature of the doctors' medical library. Waiting a few weeks, I called the medical librarian to ask about the service. She was furious. The first she had heard of the new program was when she, too, read about it in the paper. "I have no budget to buy any patient materials," she said in exasperation. "I haven't made any preparations for patient requests. There's no patient education service here. This was merely someone's idea of a good PR tactic."

COOPERATIVE CARE CENTERS: CLOSER TO THE MARK?

Another cost-saving idea studied or developed by hospitals during the past few years is the cooperative care center concept. These centers combine the features of a conventional hotel with the services of an acute care facility. They are estimated to cut hospital budgets by 40%.

How do they save money? Each patient shares his room with a cooperative care partner, usually a relative or friend who assists in the nursing care of the patient. "An educationally intensive environment can reduce post-hospital utilization—as well as cut costs," reported a 1983 Johns Hopkins University study of such programs. Hospitals took note and began to experiment with the concept.

In 1979, the first cooperative care unit was started in the New York University Medical Center. A 1983 *New York Times Magazine* article titled "A Touch of Home in Hospital Care" reported a 50% saving in nursing costs. Since then, a program called Co-op Care was launched at Vanderbilt University in Nashville; and other institutions in Milwaukee, Indianapolis, Miami, San Francisco, New York and Oregon began moving in the same direction.

Patient response has been largely positive. Fran Freedgood, a cooperative care patient, reported her co-op experience to *Family Health*: "One of my doctors had a brainstorm, and moved me into what they called the co-op care program ... My husband lives with me. We eat in a cafeteria. I'm getting lessons on pill-taking from a pharmacist. I'm being taken care of, but I feel like a grown-up again. Would you believe, they gave me back my clothes!"

LOOKING BEYOND THE HYPE

But while cooperative care centers may be closer to the mark, the question is, "Are they *on* the mark?" My sense is that most are not. Actually, there is only one sure way to test whether these new programs are for real, and whether they suit you. Go visit a hospitality hospital and a cooperative care center and note how you respond to them. Do they seem different to you? Do they feel real? Will your spirit be impoverished or enriched in such an environment? Those who visit Mother Teresa's hospital have no doubt of the sincerity of her efforts. No fancy brochures or large outlays of money are needed to prove that point. There is simply a feeling inside the clinic that tells you all you need to know about her service.

I'm not suggesting that these institutions are consciously doing something wrong, only that many may not be doing much that is good. The difference boils down to motivation. When institutional change is motivated by a genuine desire to serve patients, the result is not only upgraded services, but all sorts of secondary benefits, such as higher staff morale and increased hospital profits. But if profits are the *chief* motivation, no amount of clever marketing will disguise the fact that the new "hospitality" is being dispensed by the old hospital, taught to freshen up its image and mind its manners. When this is the case, no matter how expensive the brochures and attractive the decor, the care partner and cooperative care concepts simply will not work. Patients and family members will eventually look beyond the hype, and their resentment at what they see will erode and ultimately negate any good that initially may have flowed from the change.

If that happens, the program will inevitably fail.

BECOMING THE CHANGE

Dr. Rachel Naomi Remen, physician and author of *The Human Patient*, writes, "If technological medicine is to more fully meet human needs, both professionals and patients must be willing to examine certain fundamental assumptions we make about each other and take the risk of relating to each other in different ways. It will not be enough to simply call for the kind of change that is needed, it will be necessary for each of us to become that change."

Angelica Thieriot became the change. And although the research findings are not in from the Planetree experiment, we do know this: It is possible to provide a high quality of care without a significant increase in costs. Personnel, which is 80% of most hospital budgets, is staffed the same for the Planetree unit as for the other medical/surgical units in the hospital. While most hospital wards struggle with patient shortage and low occupancy rates, Planetree often has a waiting list, with many requests coming from outside the San Francisco area. In fact, patients and families have sometimes been known to call the unit for the names of those doctors who admit to Planetree. In this age of health care consumerism, some patients pick Planetree first, *then* the doctors who can get them there.

A look at the Planetree Patient Log shows that their confidence hasn't been misplaced. One patient wrote: "A compassionate environment was provided where I could make a learning experience out of what could have been total despair." A daughter wrote: "Being able to stay overnight was so helpful during this stressful time. I couldn't have slept if I'd been at home." A wife wrote: "Before I came here I was so worried about what would happen when I took him home. Now I know I can handle it."

In Planetree's first year of operation, the number of physicians admitting their patients to the unit increased tenfold. One doctor explains why he sends his patients there: "The patients on the Planetree Unit tend to be more involved in their own care. As a physician, this makes my job not only more pleasurable, but actually improves the quality of the health care delivered."

Nurses at this hospital have experienced high levels of professional satisfaction while working on the Planetree unit. "Planetree lets me be the kind of nurse I've always wanted to

236

be—to help people feel better, not just run around hanging IVs."

Dr. John Gamble, Chairman of the Department of Medicine, relates these findings to the future of health care in this country: "The Planetree Model Hospital Project is setting the stage for the future of hospital care. All our research and experience indicates that the incorporation of modern medicine and technology in a setting that upholds the full rights and dignity of the individual patient will add immeasurably to healing."

John C. Aird has become the change. While serving as administrator of San Jose Medical Center and, more recently, as president of its hospital consortium, he has become this country's first chief executive officer in health care to actively step forward and seek out the Planetree model for the institution he represents.

Moreover, in the specific area of care partnering, he plans to take the program beyond the San Francisco model. Patients' rooms will be designed to comfortably acccommodate the family, with ample counter space and a small counter refrigerator in each room. There will be a separate care-partner room for resting and sleeping. On Sundays, a noontime buffet will be served on the unit to welcome family members into the program.

Nurses and other staff will be hired who especially understand and support the care partner philosophy. A social worker will be assigned half-time to the unit to facilitate the care partner approach. Volunteers will be recruited and trained to serve as care partners for those without family. And care partner support group meetings will be held biweekly.

San Jose Medical Center is the first institution to adopt the Planetree approach. But it won't be the last. A continuous stream of calls come to Planetree from hospital administrators throughout the country, inquiring how Planetree resource centers and hospital units can be introduced into their institutions.

But ordinary people don't need to wait for institutions to act. We can make it happen on our own. If we can acknowledge the inner teacher who resides within our hearts, we don't have to rely on experts to usher in reform. We can become the change ourselves.

For those who feel we cannot operate alone, the POWER OF 3 offers the way. A patient can call a friend into his room and say, "Let's do something here . . . Now what was that social worker's name we liked?" Or it can be a nurse who's given up on the system—given up on administrators, on doctors, on nurses' unions, even on her own unit to solve her problems. So she picks out a patient she particularly likes, goes into his room and says, "How would you like to try this new type of program called care partnership? Do you think your sister would like to join us?" A patient can take this book to his doctor. A visitor can bring it to a nursing home friend. The initiative can be taken by anyone.

With this beginning, the POWER OF 3 can come into play. A triad can accomplish more than any one person acting alone. It can increase hospital and nursing home reform exponentially—to the POWER OF 3.

When this happens, the movement can take off. Retirement communities, housing projects, churches, synogogues can have care partner programs already in place when a resident or member enters a hospital or nursing home setting. Self-help groups can provide self-help services to members who become sick. Support groups for those who've experienced strokes, Alzheimer's, multiple sclerosis, brain injury, physical disabilities, cancer and AIDS can become care partners whenever members need hospital support.

Participants of senior companion groups and foster grandparent programs can become care partners when older friends become acutely ill. The People's Medical Society, the Gray Panthers and other patients' rights and advocacy groups can adopt this as a positive alternative to the conditions they now protest. Activists for nursing home reform, ombudsmen for long-term care, state and county commissioners on aging and health can work side by side with professionals to create a health care system where "health" and "care" mean what they say.

The moment has come for the change. Patients *can* feel better. Family members *can* find ways to externalize anxiety and pain. Professionals *can* reduce their stress. Everyone *can* share power, share responsibility, share feelings together. As friends, we *can* become good medicine for each other.

It is time to heal our institutions. Each of us can make a difference. We must make a change. This is the call for revolution.

A MODERN "ASKLEPIA"

The ancient Greeks had their *Asklepia*, a center of healing run by the priests but open to all people. Under one roof was housed a gymnasium for the well, a hospital for the ill, and a temple to serve both. In fact, people from everywhere were drawn to this temple. They believed there was so much power within its walls that to merely sleep there overnight would inspire a dream that could guide their lives. Here was a truly holistic center—one that valued the body, the mind and the spirit.

This is my dream—a modern *Asklepia*. A place that promotes caring as well as curing for patients and their families. A place where staff is supported—their bodies restored, their feelings validated, their souls renewed. A place where personal growth is encouraged for everyone involved in the promotion of healing and the preservation of wellness. In short, a place truly capable of mobilizing and directing the POWER OF 3.

What would a modern *Asklepia* be like? I can envision every institution as a "teaching hospital," but in the broadest possible sense. These would be places where patients and family members could order packets of material that explain their illnesses. Where they could keep their medical charts in their rooms, reading them at will and writing in their comments. Where their ideas and perceptions, and those of their family, would be valued. Where they, as the persons most affected by the healing process, could set up healing environments specific to *their* needs, interests and comforts. *Where patients could quite literally become teachers*, leading case conferences when appropriate and conducting medical and nursing rounds.

In such a hospital, patients could choose or be assigned to a primary physician and a primary nurse. This team would look to their patients for daily, scheduled feedback on their performance. Patients would feel comfortable saying what it felt like to be catheterized, given biopsy results, diagnosed as having cancer. Family members would say if they felt rushed or misunderstood. Conversely, staff would speak up too. They would disclose what it was like to deliver painful news, disconnect respirators, deal with treatment failures. In the *Askelpia*, everyone could laugh, cry and hope.

Patients, family members, staff would have opportunities

240

to submit the name of anyone who had shown "outstanding healing leadership and care." Such nominations would be received by a hospital committee made up of professionals and community members. From time to time, this committee would make humanitarian awards.

Space and leadership would be provided for aerobic and yoga classes, meditation rooms and regular massage for patients, family members and staff.

When new buildings were constructed or old structures redone, they would be designed with patients' emotional and spiritual needs in mind. The use of color, the arts, the natural environment would all be taken into account. Relying more on forethought than money, planners would create hospitals that would look and feel more like universities than like penitentiaries.

Ultimately, hospitals could once again become symbolic temples. They could grow into places of such physical and spiritual beauty that people everywhere would be drawn to them—to eat lunches on their grounds, spend Sunday afternoons inside their foyers. And there they could dream the dreams that would guide their lives.

I'm convinced it can—and will—happen. But something else must happen first. People inside and outside hospital walls must decide that any other form of health care is unacceptable. Then they must make the commitment—in their hearts and in their minds —to work together to make it work.

BECAUSE THEY ARE RIGHT

Dr. Jean Shinoda Bolen, a psychiatrist and Jungian analyst, lectures to audiences across the country on the principles of synchronicity in making life-choices. She says this: "Does your choice have heart? If your decision is based on greed, ambition, fear or duty, you may regret the course you've taken all your life. If your choice has heart, the universe will open doors for you and you will find meaning and fulfillment in everything you do. It's all very simple, but you must be very careful. One course weakens you, the other course makes you strong."

There are many reasons why hospital reform can't happen. Too costly. Too much staff time required. Patients not interested. Health workers apathetic. But there is an important answer to these objections—one we forget as we allow ourselves to be deflected by the "conventional wisdom" of the past or the "realistic limitations" of the present.

At a conference called for the opening of the Planetree Unit in 1985, reporters from the *New York Times*, *The Boston Globe* and other major newspapers came loaded with questions.

"Do you expect doctors to accept an 'open chart' philosophy?"

"Do you expect to maintain the standard patient/nurse ratio?"

"Do you expect to increase the hospital occupancy rate?"

"Do you expect the Planetree model to be more cost-effective?"

Reporters and photographers stood up at their chairs, pencils racing across small note pads clutched in their hands, flash bulbs exploding in short bursts of blinding light. The panel member who was about to speak was the highly respected Albert R. Jonsen, Ph.D., Professor of Ethics and Medicine and Chief of the Division of Medical Ethics, School of Medicine, University of California, San Francisco. Dr.

Jonsen looked out at the assembled media and waited for the room to grow quiet. Then he gave them their answer.

"What we are talking about here are values," he said. "Granting autonomy to patients is valued here. And these values affect the entire institution. In this context, it is simply enough to do things because they are right."

23 Lark Court
Larkspur, CA 94939
October 1, 1990

Dear Readers,

I'm very interested in how you've created a care partnership and utilized the POWER OF 3 in your hospital or nursing home. If you would care to write to me, I would welcome your ideas and suggestions for a Care Partner Newsletter.

You may also wish to recommend someone within your hospital or nursing home—a nurse, doctor, orderly, patient or family member—for a humanitarian award in health care. Please send the person's name, title, institution and address. Then describe in a page or less why you think this person should be honored as an outstanding leader in the field of "healing and care." Or you may wish to submit your ideas for our modern *Asklepia*, or recommend a particular institution that is striving for these ideals.

Please enclose a self-addressed stamped envelope if you care to receive our first newsletter.

If you need assistance in starting a Care Partner Program in your institution, club, church or neighborhood, you can contact me at the address above.

I support you in your interest and your efforts. I'm convinced that when we join with others of like minds, we can create extraordinary change. Together we *can* bring "caring" back into health "care."

Sincerely yours,

Mary Dale Scheller, M.S.W.

245

APPENDICES

Appendix 1

HEALTH RESOURCE CENTERS/
CONSUMERS' MEDICAL LIBRARIES

The Center for Medical
Consumers
237 Thompson Street
New York, NY 10012
(212) 674-7105

- Medical Health Library
- Biweekly Radio Show
- Monthly Newsletter
- Self-Help Group Referrals
- Publications

Health Education Center
200 Ross Street
Pittsburgh, PA 15219
(412) 392-3160

- Health Consultants
- Literature Reviews
- Training
- Publications

Health Education Center
of the Kaiser-Permanente
Medical Care Program
3772 Howe Street
Oakland, CA 94611
(415) 428-6569

- Consumers' Health Library
- Films, Audio/Video Tapes
- Health Education Programs
- Support Group Information
- Community Service Referral
- Self-Care Displays
  & Information
- Children's Section
- TV and Study Booths
- Health Store

Healthworks for Women
Mt. Zion Hospital
1600 Divisadero Street
San Francisco, CA 94115
(415) 885-7710

- Consumers' Health Library
- Physician & Community
  Referrals
- Classes
- Newsletter

247

Planetree Health Resource
Center
2040 Webster Street
San Francisco, CA 94115
(415) 346-4636

- Consumers' Health Library
- Bookstore
- Reference Center
- National Information/
  Reference
- Health Information By Mail
- Personally Prepared
  Bibliographies
- Self-Help Resources
- Audio/Video Tapes
- Newsletter

People's Medical Society
14 East Minor Street
Emmaus, PA 18049
(215) 967-2136

- Health Library
- Bimonthly Newsletter
- Publications
- Local Organizing/
  Consumer Advocacy

The Sutter Resource
1006 21st Street
Sacramento, CA 95814
(916) 447-4858

- Consumers' Health Library
- Classes
- Medical Information Search
- Community Service Referrals
- Personally Prepared
  Bibliographies

Appendix 2

PATIENT'S BILL OF RIGHTS

The American Hospital Association presents a Patient's Bill of Rights with the expectation that observance of these rights will contribute to more effective patient care and greater satisfaction for the patient, his physician, and the hospital organization. Further, the Association presents these rights in the expectation that they will be supported by the hospital on behalf of its patients, as an integral part of the healing process. It is recognized that a personal relationship between the physician and the patient is essential for the provision of proper medical care. The traditional physician-patient relationship takes on a new dimension when care is rendered within an organizational structure. Legal precedent has established that the institution itself also has a responsibility to the patient. It is in recognition of these factors that these rights are affirmed.

1. The patient has the right to considerate and respectful care.
2. The patient has the right to obtain from his physician complete current information concerning his diagnosis, treatment, and prognosis in terms the patient can be reasonably expected to understand. When it is not medically advisable to give such information to the patient, the information should be made available to an appropriate person in his behalf. He has the right to know by name, the physician responsible for coordinating his care.
3. The patient has the right to receive from his physician information necessary to give informed consent prior to the start of any procedure and/or treatment. Except in emergencies, such information for informed consent, should include but not necessarily be limited to the specific procedure and/or treatment, the medically significant risks involved, and the probable duration of incapacitation. Where medically significant alternatives for care or treatment exist, or when the patient requests information concerning medical alternatives, the patient has the right to such information. The patient also has the right to know the name of the person responsible for the procedures and/or treatment.

4. The patient has the right to refuse treatment to the extent permitted by law, and to be informed of the medical consequences of his action.

5. The patient has the right to every consideration of his privacy concerning his own medical care program. Case discussion, consultation, examination, and treatment are confidential and should be conducted discreetly. Those not directly involved in his care must have the permission of the patient to be present.

6. The patient has the right to expect that all communications and records pertaining to his care should be treated as confidential.

7. The patient has the right to expect that within its capacity a hospital must make reasonable response to the request of a patient for services. The hospital must provide evaluation, service, and/or referral as indicated by the urgency of the case. When medically permissible a patient may be transferred to another facility only after he has received complete information and explanation concerning the needs for and alternatives to such a transfer. The institution to which the patient is to be transferred must first have accepted the patient for transfer.

8. The patient has the right to obtain information as to any relationship of his hospital to other health care and educational institutions insofar as his care is concerned. The patient has the right to obtain information as to the existence of any professional relationships among individuals, by name, who are treating him.

9. The patient has the right to be advised if the hospital proposes to engage in or perform human experimentation affecting his care or treatment. The patient has the right to refuse to participate in such research projects.

10. The patient has the right to expect reasonable continuity of care. He has the right to know in advance what appointment times and physicians are available and where. The patient has the right to expect that the hospital will provide a mechanism whereby he is informed by his physician or a delegate of the physician of the patient's continuing health care requirements following discharge.

11. The patient has the right to examine and receive an explanation of his bill regardless of source of payment.

12. The patient has the right to know what hospital rules and regulations apply to his conduct as a patient.

No catalogue of rights can guarantee for the patient the kind of treatment he has a right to expect. A hospital has many functions to perform, including the prevention and treatment of disease, the education of both health professionals and the patients, and the conduct of clinical research. All these activities must be conducted with an overriding concern for the patient, and, above all, the recognition of his dignity as a human being. Success in achieving this recognition assures success in the defense of the rights of the patient.

To receive your own copy of the "The Patient's Bill of Rights" contact:
1. the social worker in your hospital
2. your county or state Department of Social Services
3. your county or state Department of Health
4. the American Hospital Association, 840 N. Lakeshore Dr., Chicago, Illinois, 60611 • (312) 280-6000
5. Concern for Dying, 250 West 57th St., New York, New York, 10107 • (212) 246-6962

Appendix 3

PATIENT'S RIGHTS IN A NURSING HOME

Most state departments of health publish statements of patient rights in nursing homes in their respective states. These usually provide for rights similar to those guaranteed by the California Department of Health Services listed below:

Each person admitted to a nursing home has the following rights, among others:

A. To be fully informed, as evidenced by the patient's written acknowledgement prior to or at the time of admission and during the stay, of these rights and of all rules and regulations governing patient conduct.

B. To be fully informed prior to or at the time of admission and during the stay of services available in the facility, and of related charges including any charges for services not covered by the facility's basic per diem rate or not covered under Titles XVIII or XIX of the Social Security Act.

C. To be fully informed by a physician of his or her medical condition, unless medically contraindicated, and to be afforded the opportunity to participate in the planning of his or her medical treatment and to refuse to participate in experimental research.

D. To refuse treatment to the extent permitted by law and to be informed of the medical consequences of such refusal.

E. To be transferred or discharged only for medical reasons or for his or her welfare or that of other patients or for nonpayment for his or her stay; to be given reasonable advance notice to ensure orderly transfer or discharge. Such actions must be documented in his or her health record.

F. To be encouraged and assisted throughout his or her stay to exercise his or her rights as a patient and as a citizen, and to this end to voice grievances and recommend changes in policies and services to facility staff and/or outside representatives of his or her choice free from restraint, interference, coercion, discrimination, or reprisal.

G. To manage his or her personal financial affairs or to be given at least quarterly accounting of financial transactions made on his or her behalf should the facility accept his or her written delegation of the responsibility subject to the provisions of the law.

H. To be free from mental and physical abuse, and to be free from chemical and (except in emergencies) physical restraints, except as authorized in writing by a physician for a specified and limited period of time or when necessary to protect the patient from injury to himself or herself or to others.

I. To be assured confidential treatment of his or her personal and medical records, and to approve or refuse their release to any individual outside the facility except in the case of his or her transfer to another health facility or as required by law or third party payment contract..

J. To be treated with consideration, respect, and full recognition of his or her dignity and individuality including privacy in treatment and care for his or her personal needs.

K. Not to be required to perform services for the facility that are not included for therapeutic purposes in his or her plan of care.

L. To associate and communicate privately with persons of his or choice and to send and receive his or her personal mail unopened unless medically contraindicated.

M. To meet with and participate in the activities of social, religious, and community groups at his or her discretion unless medically contraindicated.

N. To retain and use his or her personal clothing and possessions as space permits unless to do so would infringe upon the rights of other patients and unless medically contraindicated.

O. If married, to be assured privacy for visits by his or her spouse, and, if both are patients in the facility, to be permitted to share a room unless medically contraindicated.

P. To have daily visiting hours established.

Q. To have members of the clergy admitted at the request of the patient or person responsible at any time.

R. To allow relatives or persons responsible to visit critically ill patients at any time unless medically contraindicated.

S. To be allowed privacy for visits with family, friends, clergy, social workers, or for professional or business purposes.

T. To have reasonable access to telephones—both to make and receive confidential calls.

To receive a copy of your state's "Patient's Rights in a Nursing Home" contact:
1. the social worker or administrator of your nursing home
2. your county or state Department of Social Services
3. your county or state Department of Health
4. your county Area Agency on Aging or state Department on Aging
5. your county or state Ombudsman for Nursing Home Care

To receive a copy of the State of California's "A Consumer Guide to Nursing Homes" and your own copy of California's "Patient's Rights in a Nursing Home" contact:

> State of California
> Department of Health Services
> Licensing and Certification Division
> 714 "P" Street
> Sacramento, CA 95814

Appendix 4

STATE LAWS GIVING PATIENTS THE RIGHT TO ACCESS MEDICAL RECORDS

STATE STATUTE	ACCESS TO RECORDS: DRS.	HOSP.	RIGHT TO INSPECT	RIGHT TO COPY	*LIMITS./ SPECS.
ALABAMA, Code tit 22, §50-62 (1975)					X
ALASKA Stat, §47. 30.260 (1979) §18. 23.065 (Supp.)	X	X	X	X	X
ARIZONA Rev. Stat, §36.509 (1974) & §36.568.01 (Supp. 1979)					X
CALIFORNIA Evid. Code §1158 (Supp. 1980); Welf. & Inst. Code §5328 (Supp 1980); 53 Cal. Op. Att'y Gen §151; Health & Safety Code §§25250–25258, Div. 20	X	X	X	X	X
COLORADO Rev. Stat. §25-1-801-803 (Supp. 1978) & §27-10-120 (1973) as amended (1978)	X	X	X	X	X
CONNECTICUT Gen. Stat. Ann. §4-104 (1969) & §17-206i(b) (Supp.1980)		X	X	X	X
DELAWARE Code tit. 16, §5161(a)(7) (1974)					X
D.C. Code §21-562 (1973) §6-1611 (Supp. VII 1980)					X
FLORIDA Stat. Ann. §455.241 (Supp. 1980) §394.459 (1973), as amended 1979, & §395.202	X	X	X	X	X
GEORGIA Code Ann. §88.502.12 (1979) as amended 1979					X

STATE LAWS GIVING PATIENTS THE RIGHT TO ACCESS MEDICAL RECORDS

STATE STATUTE	ACCESS TO RECORDS: DRS.	HOSP.	RIGHT TO INSPECT	RIGHT TO COPY	*LIMITS./ SPECS.
HAWAII Rev. Stat. §662-57 (1976) & §334-5 (1976)	X	X		X	X
IDAHO Code §66-348 (Supp. 1979)					X
ILLINOIS Ann. Stat. Ch. 51, §§71, 72, 73 Supp. (1980) & Ch. 91 1/2 §804, Supp. (1980)	X	X	X	X	X
INDIANA Code §34-3-15. 5-4 (1976) & §16-14-1. 6-8 Cum Supp. (1979)		X	X	X	X
KANSAS Stat. Ann. §59-2931 (1976)					X
KENTUCKY Rev. Stat. §210.235 (1975)					X
LOUISIANA Rev. Stat. §§40:1299.96, 40:2013.3 & 40:2014.1 (West 1977 & Supp. 1980)	X	X		X	X
MAINE Rev. Stat. Ann. tit. 34, §1-B (1978), as amended 1979 and tit. 22, §1711 (1980)		X		X	X
MARYLAND Ann. Code art. 48A, §490 C (1979); 1978 Md. Laws, Ch. 815					X
MASSACHUSETTS Ann. Laws Ch. 111, §70 (1975) as amended 1975, Ch. 111,§70E (Supp.1980) & Ch. 123, §36 (1975)		X	X	X	X

STATE LAWS GIVING PATIENTS THE RIGHT TO ACCESS MEDICAL RECORDS

STATE STATUTE	ACCESS TO RECORDS: DRS.	HOSP.	RIGHT TO INSPECT	RIGHT TO COPY	*LIMITS./ SPECS.
MICHIGAN Stat. Ann. §14.800 (748) (1976) & Cum. Supp. (1980); §14.15 (2639) (Cum. Supp.1980)	X	X	X		X
MINNESOTA Stat. Ann. §144.335 (Supp. 1980)	X	X			X
MISSISSIPPI Code Ann. §41-9-65 (1973) & §41-21-97, Supp. (1979)		X			X
MISSOURI Ann. Stat. §§202.195, 202.197 (Supp. 1980)					X
NEBRASKA Bishop Clarkson Memorial Hospital v. Reserve Life Insurance Co., 350F. 2d 1006 (8th Cir. 1965)		X	X	X	X
NEVADA Rev. Stat. §629.061 (1977)	X	X	X	X	
NEW JERSEY Stat. Ann. §30:4-24.3, (Supp. 1979) & §2A:82-42 (1976)		X	X		X
NEW YORK Mental Hyg. Law §33-13 (1978), amended (1979); Rules of the N.Y. State Board of Regents Relating to Definitions of Unprofessional Conduct (1977) 29.2 (a) (7): 29.1 (b) (13)	X			X	X
NORTH CAROLINA Gen. Stat. §122-8.1 (1974), as amended 1979					X

STATE LAWS GIVING PATIENTS THE RIGHT TO ACCESS MEDICAL RECORDS

STATE STATUTE	ACCESS TO RECORDS:		RIGHT TO INSPECT	RIGHT TO COPY	*LIMITS./ SPECS.
	DRS.	HOSP.			
NORTH DAKOTA Cent. Code §25-03. 1-43 (1978) & §25-16-07 (1978)					X
OHIO Rev. Code Ann. §5123.89 (Supp.1979)		X			X
OKLAHOMA Stat. Ann. tit. 76, §19, (Supp. 1979)	X	X	X	X	X
OREGON Rev. Stat. §§192.525, 192.530 (1977) & §441.810 (1977)	X	X		X	X
PENNSYLVANIA Stat. Ann. tit. 50, §4602 (1969)					X
SOUTH DAKOTA Comp. Laws Ann. §§27A-12-28, 27A-12-28 & 24-12-15 (1976 & Supp. 1979)		X		X	X
TENNESSEE Code Ann. §53-1322 (1977) & §33-306 (1977), as amended 1978		X			X
TEXAS Rev. Civ. Stat. Ann. art. 5547-87 (1958) as amended 1979		X			X
UTAH Code Ann. §78-25-25 (1977) & §64-7-50 (1978)	X	X			X
VERMONT Stat. Ann. tit. 18, §7103 (1968)					X
VIRGINIA Code §8.01-413 (1977) §2.1-342 (1976) as amended 1980, §37.1-84.1(8) (1976) & §37.1-230, (Supp. 1980)	X	X	X	X	X

STATE LAWS GIVING PATIENTS THE RIGHT TO ACCESS MEDICAL RECORDS

STATE STATUTE	ACCESS TO RECORDS: DRS.	HOSP.	RIGHT TO INSPECT	RIGHT TO COPY	*LIMITS./ SPECS.
WASHINGTON Rev. Code Ann. §71.05.390 (1975), as amended 1979					X
WEST VIRGINIA Code §27-3-1 (1980)					X
WISCONSIN Stat. Ann. §804.10 (4) (1977), §908.03 (6m) (b) (Supp. 1979), §51.30(4)(d)(3) (Supp.1979); 1979 Wis. Laws, Ch. 221, to become Wis. Stat Ann. §§146-81-83	X	X	X	X	X
WYOMING Stat. Ann. §25-3-126 (1977)					X

* Certain specifications, such as provisions for or exceptions to psychiatric or mental health records. Access may be limited to certain requirements set in statute, such as copy of hospital record available only after discharge or access limited to doctor's judgment concerning whether information would be harmful to patient.

Sources:
Medical Records: Getting Yours: A Consumer's Guide to Obtaining Your Medical Records. Health Research Group, 2000 "P" Street N.W., Suite 708, Washington, D.C. 20036

Guidelines for Implementation of AB 610: Patient Access to Medical Records. California Medical Record Association, Inc., Oct. 1982

Appendix 5

HOSPITAL MUSIC LIST

Steve Bergman, *Soothing Lullabies*, Sweet Baby Dreams, 220 Dela Vina, Monterey, CA 93940 (For expectant mothers, crying babies and children. Three tapes: *Lullabies from around the World, Slumberland, Sweet Baby Dreams*. Flutes, guitar, string orchestra and synthesizers combine with soothing sounds of birds, crickets and heartbeats.)

Ron Dexter, *Golden Voyages*, Vols. 1-4, Awakening Productions, 4132 Tuller Avenue, Culver City, CA 90230 (New Age music blended with water, birds, and woodland sounds.)

The Environment Series, Syntonic Research Series, Atlantic Label, (Environmental sounds from the seashore and countryside.)

Steven Halpern, *Spectrum Suite* (HS 770), Halpern Sounds, P.O. Box 720, Palo Alto, CA 94302 (Synthesizer and flute provide meditative sounds corresponding to energy and healing centers of the body. Other compositions include: *Comfort Zone, Starborn Suite, Zodiac Suite*, and *Eastern Peace*.)

Georgia Kelly, *Tarashanti*, Heru Records, P.O. Box 954, Topanga, CA. 90290 (Music for harp and flute. Other compositions include: *Sea Peace, Birds of Paradise*, and *Ancient Echoes*.)

Michael McQuilkin and Richard Schoenherz, *Open Channel*, One Life Music, 139 Humboldt Ave, San Rafael, CA. 94901 (Synthesizers, electronic percussions, tablas and Tibetan bells "open the channel" for relaxation, healing and love.)

Daniel Kobialka, *Timeless Motion*, Li-Sem Enterprises, Inc., 490 El Camino Real, Suite 215, Belmont, CA 94002 (New Age compositions and a slow extended version of Pachelbel's Canon in D.)

John LoGiudici and Dave Parrett, *High Hopes*, Search Party Music, P.O. Box 40207, San Francisco, CA 94140 (Spanish, steel-string and electric guitars combined with piano and synthesizer.)

Ray Lynch, *Deep Breakfast*, Ray Lynch Productions, P.O. Box 252, San Rafael, CA 94915 (Upbeat and positive music. A "deep breakfast of pure sunlight.")

Relax with the Classics, The Lind Institute, San Francisco, CA., (Baroque masterpieces scientifically selected and sequenced for relaxation.)

Mike Rowland, *Fairy Ring*, Narada Distributing, 207 E. Buffalo, Milwaukee, WI 53202 (Gentle piano and synthesized strings.)

Joseph and Nathan Segal, *Songs from a Course in Miracles*, Birds of Wisdom Records, 2031 Union Street, San Francisco, CA 94123 (A Jewish rabbi and cantor add their voices and music to lyrics taken from *A Course in Miracles*. Another album of beautiful music put to biblical scripture is *From You I Receive*.)

A Treasury of Gregorian Chants, Vol. I and II, Monks of the Abbey St. Thomas, VOX Records.

George Winston, *Autumn*, Windham Hill Records, P.O. Box 9388, Stanford, CA. 94305 (Relaxing piano solos. Other albums include: *Winter* and *Winter into Spring*.)

GUIDED IMAGERY TAPES

Louise Hay, *Self-Healing: Creating Your Health*, Hay House, 3029 Wilshire Blvd. #206, Santa Monica, CA 90404 (Lecture and meditation designed to help the listener let go of negative emotions. Also available are tapes specific to AIDS and cancer.)

Dr. Emmett Miller, *Healing Journey*, SOURCE, P.O. Box W, Stanford, CA. 94305 (Combination of body relaxation and mental imagery. Other tapes include: *Successful Surgery and Recovery: Conditioning Mind and Body*; *Rainbow Butterfly* with Georgia Kelly; and *Letting Go of Stress* with Steven Halpern.)

Dr. Martin Rossman, *Healing Yourself,* Insight Publishing, Box 2070, Mill Valley, CA 94942 (This and a six-cassette series follow information from Rossman's book, *Healing Yourself: A Step-By-Step Program for Better Health through Imagery.*)

Katherine Tessner and Tina Dungan, *Breaking the Silence: A Soothing Meditation for the Child Within,* A.C.A.T., 1275 4th St., Santa Monica, CA. 90404 (A blend of ocean sounds, harp and piano with affirmations that help with letting go of fears and worries. Originally designed for children of alcoholics, but helpful to anyone suffering from emotional hurts.)

Dr. Bernard Siegel, *Exceptional Cancer Patients: Guided Imagery and Meditation,* ECAP Office, 2 Church St. S, New Haven, CT 06519 (To background music of Pachelbel's Canon in D, imagery is employed through balloon rides and magic playgrounds to heal the child within. Includes Dr. Siegel's personal approach to working with patients in coma, asleep or under anesthesia.)

Appendix 6

EXAMPLE OF A LIVING WILL

To my family, my physician, my lawyer and all others whom it may concern:

Death is as much a reality as birth, growth, maturity and old age—it is the one certainty of life. If the time comes when I can no longer take part in decisions for my own future, let this statement stand as an expression of my wishes and directions, while I am still of sound mind.

If at such a time the situation should arise in which there is no reasonable expectation of my recovery from extreme physical or mental disability, I direct that I be allowed to die and not be kept alive by medications, artificial means or "heroic measures." I do, however, ask that medication be mercifully administered to me to alleviate suffering even though this may shorten my remaining life.

This statement is made after careful consideration and is in accordance with my strong convictions and beliefs. I want the wishes and directions here expressed carried out to the extent permitted by law. Insofar as they are not legally enforceable, I hope that those to whom this Will is addressed will regard themselves as morally bound by these provisions.

Signed ——————————————

Date ——————————————

Witness ——————————————

Witness ——————————————

Copies of this request have been given to

——————————————

——————————————

——————————————

For further information contact: Concern For Dying
250 West 57th Street
New York, New York 10107
(212) 246-6962

263

Appendix 7

DEFINITIONS, ADVANTAGES AND DRAWBACKS OF: LIVING WILLS/
NATURAL DEATH ACTS / DURABLE POWER OF ATTORNEY ACTS /
CONSERVATORSHIPS /FAMILY CONSENT ACTS

LIVING WILL—A document which enables an individual, while competent, to give his/her directions for treatment decisions during terminal illness, including the withholding or withdrawal of life-support systems.

Advantages:

- Any person, without restriction, can specify ahead of time how he/she wants to be treated in regard to life-sustaining treatments. Such specifications usually cover the determination to use or refrain from using (1) a ventilator for performing respiration, (2) an IV system for providing fluids and medicine, (3) a naso-gastric tube for providing nutrition, and (4) any other aggressive treatment directed at delaying death rather than providing comfort.
- A living will offers guidance to doctors and family members when the patient can no longer participate in his or her care.

Drawbacks:

- Living wills have no legal weight. Health professionals are not required to follow them. Professionals who do follow them are not protected from civil or criminal suits.
- There are no legal penalites for their misuse, e.g., their destruction or concealment, the use of forgery, or the disregard of their instructions.

NATURAL DEATH ACT—State legislation which gives a competent adult the legal right under circumstances spelled out in the legislation to sign a written directive instructing his/her physician how to direct treatment at the end of his/her life. Some states refer to this legislation as a Right to Die Act. Others use other names.

DIRECTIVE TO MY PHYSICIAN—A written document similar to a living will, but with its instructions precisely spelled out and its authority backed by state legislation.

Advantages:
- Backed by legal sanctions, most natural death acts offer safeguards against the drawbacks experienced with living wills, which have no state laws behind them.

Drawbacks:
- In an attempt to protect those patients susceptible to signing such documents prematurely, most state statutes set up rigorous requirements that patients must meet.
- Each state differs in its definition of and penalties for misuse of the document.
- With no uniformity in state laws, if one is stricken outside one's home state, the out-of-state document might not be honored.

DURABLE POWER OF ATTORNEY—A state law allowing a person (principal) to designate another individual to make decisions for him/her should he/she become incapacitated at some future time. ("Durable" means beyond the conventional power of attorney. A "springing" durable power of attorney "springs" into use *only* if the principal becomes incapacitated.)

Advantages:
- The designated decision maker can be kept current with up-to-date medical information and procedures, thus guarding against a situation where outdated instructions written in the past restrict responsible decision making.
- The patient gets to pick his/her representative.
- The durable power of attorney does not require any action by the courts.

Drawbacks:
- Although the representative is picked by the patient, the patient is not the decision maker.
- The durable power of attorney does not deal with potential problems of conflict-of-interest, e.g., in cases where the representative is a debtor, creditor or heir.
- Most durable power of attorneys do not specify what will happen if the representative is temporarily or permanently unable or un-

338

willing to serve, e.g., out of town or seriously ill when the decision must be made.

- The durable power of attorney may not hold up in court unless the state legislation specifically includes health care decisions.

DURABLE POWER OF ATTORNEY IN HEALTH CARE DECISIONS—A state law specifically extending durable power of attorney to health care decisions.

Advantages:

- In cases where the requirements of the law have been met, the legislation should hold up in court for health care decisions.

(However, all the other advantages and drawbacks of the generic durable power of attorney are present in this form.)

CONSERVATORSHIP—A court action where one person is decreed incompetent and another is designated to make all decisions on his/her behalf. (Some states use different names, such as guardianship, curatorship, or custodianship. However the court proceedings are much the same.)

Advantages:

- In health care decisions, a conservatorship provides for a legally authorized decision maker when no durable power of attorney exists.
- An early conservatorship may be desirable when a family dispute (and subsequent litigation) can be predicted over the validity of a durable power of attorney. In such case, a court proceeding of some sort will be necessary anyway.
- A conservatorship is necessary when no one is able or willing to serve as the patient's designated decision maker with a durable power of attorney.

Drawbacks:

- Court proceedings are usually lengthy, costly and sometimes emotionally draining.
- Although the court is held responsible for appointing a conservator who will serve in the conservatee's "best interest," the appointee may not be the person whom the patient or the family members would have chosen.

FAMILY CONSENT ACT—A state law that gives a specific family member the right to make health care decisions for a relative who is in a coma, or in some cases, in the last stages of a terminal illness. Each statute is different in its requirements, including the specifications of which family member becomes the decision maker.

Advantages:
- In states with this legislation, a patient would not have to prepare a durable power of attorney before the time of incapacitation nor would a family member have to go to court to secure the legal right to make health care decisions for the patient.
- This legislation codifies what is often done informally in hospitals where no durable power of attorney exists.

Drawbacks:
- With most of the laws, the actual designation of the decision maker is often unclear or difficult to implement.
- There are rarely procedures set forth to handle disputes within a family, when consensus is not achieved.

For information on legislation or forms specific to your state contact:

1. The Department of Social Services in your hospital or nursing home
2. Your county or state Department of Social Service or Department of Health
3. Concern for Dying
   250 West 57th Street
   New York, New York 10107
   (212) 246-6962

Appendix 8

TION PROVIDING FOR:

	DURABLE POWER OF ATTORNEY	DURABLE POWER OF ATTORNEY FOR HEALTH CARE	FAMILY CONSENT ACTS
	ALABAMA Code § 26-1-2 (1975)		
A §§ 2.010 - 0 (1986)	ALASKA Stat. §§ 13.26.325 & 13.26.330		
ARIZONA Rev. Stat. Ann. §§ 36-3201 - 3210 (1985)	ARIZONA Rev. Stat. Ann. §§ 14-5501 & 5502		
ARKANSAS Ark. Acts 713 (1987)	ARKANSAS Stat. Ann. §§ 58-701 - 704 (1983)		ARKANSAS Stat. § 82-363 (1976)
CALIFORNIA Health & Safety Code §§ 7185 - 7195 (1976)	CALIFORNIA Civil Code §§ 2400-2407 & §§ 2410-2423	CALIFORNIA Civ. Code § 2500 (1987)	
COLORADA Rev. Stat. §§ 15-18-101 - 113 (1985)	COLORADO *		
CONNECTICUT Gen. Stat. §§ 19a-570 - 575 (1985)	CONNECTICUT Gen. Stat. Ann. § 45-69o		
DELAWARE Code Ann. tit 16, §§ 2501-2509 (1982)	DELAWARE Code Ann. Title 12, §§ 4901- 4905		

STATE LEGISLATION PROVIDING FOR:

NATURAL DEATH ACTS/ RIGHT TO DIE ACTS	DURABLE POWER OF ATTORNEY	DURABLE POWER OF ATTORNEY FOR HEALTH CARE	FAMILY CONSENT ACTS
D.C. Code Ann. §§ 6-2421- 2430 (1982)	D.C. Code Ann. Title 21, §§ 2081-2085 (1987 supp.)		
FLORIDA Stat. Ann. §§ 765.01 - .15 (1984)	FLORIDA Statutes §§ 709.08 (1983)		FLORIDA Stat.Ch. 84-85, § 765.0 (1984)
GEORGIA Code Ann. §§ 31-32-1 - 12 (1984)	GEORGIA Code Ann. §§ 10-6-3 - 10-6-36		GEORGIA Code § 31-9-1 (1982)
HAWAII Rev. Stat. §§ 327D-1 - 27 (1986)	HAWAII Rev. Stat. §§ 560:5-501 & 5-502		
IDAHO Code §§ 39-4501 - 4508 (1977)	IDAHO §§ 15-5-501 - 5-507		IDAHO Code § 39-4303 (1985)
ILLINOIS Rev. Stat. ch 110 1/2 §§ 701 (1984)	ILLINOIS Rev. Stat. ch. 110 1/2, § 11a-3	ILLINOIS Stat. ch. 110 1/2 §§ 804-1 - 12 (1987)	
INDIANA Code Ann. §§ 16-8-11-1 - 22 (1985)	INDIANA Code Ann. § 30-2-1.5-1		

STATE LEGISLATION PROVIDING FOR:

NATURAL DEATH ACTS/ RIGHT TO DIE ACTS	DURABLE POWER OF ATTORNEY	DURABLE POWER OF ATTORNEY FOR HEALTH CARE	FAMILY CONSENT ACTS
IOWA Code Ann. §§ 144A.1 - .11 (1985)	IOWA Code Ann. §§ 63.705 & 706		IOWA Code Ch. 144A.1- 144A.12 (1985)
KANSAS Stat. Ann. §§ 65-28,101 - 28,109 (1979)	KANSAS Stat. Ann. §§ 58-610 - 58-617		
	KENTUCKY Rev. Stat. Ann. § 386.093		
LOUISIANA Rev. Stat. Ann. §§ 40:1299.58.1- .10 (1984)	LOUISIANA Civ. Code Ann., Article 3027		LOUISIANA Rev. Stat. Ann. tit 40 § 1299-58.5 (A) (H.B.795 1985)
MAINE Rev. Stat. Ann. tit. 22, §§ 2921-2931 (1985)	MAINE * Rev. Stat. Ann. tit. 18-A, § 5-501		MAINE Rev. Stat. Ann. tit 24, § 2905 (1985)
MARYLAND Health-Gen. Code Ann. §§ 5-601 - 614 (1985)	MARYLAND Code Ann. §§ 13-601 - 13-603		MARYLAND Ann. Code (Health Gen) § 20-107(d) (1984)
	MASSACHUSETTS Gen. Laws Ann., Ch 201B, §§ 1-6		

STATE LEGISLATION PROVIDING FOR:

NATURAL DEATH ACTS/ RIGHT TO DIE ACTS	DURABLE POWER OF ATTORNEY	DURABLE POWER OF ATTORNEY FOR HEALTH CARE	FAMILY CONSENT ACTS
	MICHIGAN Stat. Ann. § 27.5495 (1980)		
	MINNESOTA Stat. Ann. §§ 524.5-501 & 502 (1982)		
MISSISSIPPI Code Ann. §§ 41-41-101 - 121 (1984)	MISSISSIPPI Code Ann. §§ 87-3-1 - 97-3-17		MISSISSIPPI Code Ann. § 41 - 41-3 (1985)
MISSOURI Stat. Ann. §§ 459.010-.055 (1985)	MISSOURI Rev. Stat §§ 486.550 - 486.595		
MONTANA Code Ann. §§ 50-9-101-104, 111, 202-206 (1985)			
	NEBRASKA Rev. Stat. §§ 30-2662 & 2663		
NEVADA Rev. Stat. §§ 449.540-.690 (1977)	NEVADA Rev. Stat. §§ 111.460 & 111.470	NEVADA Statutes, ch. 396 (1987) Nev. Rev. Stat. §§ 111.470 (1987)	

STATE LEGISLATION PROVIDING FOR:

NATURAL DEATH ACTS/ RIGHT TO DIE ACTS	DURABLE POWER OF ATTORNEY	DURABLE POWER OF ATTORNEY FOR HEALTH CARE	FAMILY CONSENT ACTS
NEW HAMPSHIRE Rev. Stat. Ann. §§ 137-H:1-16 (1985)	NEW HAMPSHIRE Rev. Stat. Ann. § 506:6		
	NEW JERSEY ** Stat. Ann. § 46:2B-8 (West Supp. 1983-84)		
NEW MEXICO Stat. Ann. §§ 24-7-1-11 (1977)	NEW MEXICO Stat. Ann. §§ 45-5-501 & 502		NEW MEXICO Stat.Ann. § 24-7-5 amended S.B. 15 (1984)
	NEW YORK [Gen. Oblig.] Law 5-1502 & 5-1601 (1978)		
NORTH CAROLINA Gen. Stat. §§ 90-320-322 (1977)	NORTH CAROLINA * Gen. Stat. §§ 32A-1 - 32A-4		NORTH CAROLINA Gen.Stat. § 90-322 (b) amended S.B.240(1983)
	NORTH DAKOTA Cent. Code §§ 30.1-30-01 & 02		
	OHIO Rev. Code Ann. §§ 1337.09 & 1337.091		

STATE LEGISLATION PROVIDING FOR:

NATURAL DEATH ACTS/ RIGHT TO DIE ACTS	DURABLE POWER OF ATTORNEY	DURABLE POWER OF ATTORNEY FOR HEALTH CARE	FAMILY CONSENT ACTS
OKLAHOMA Stat. Ann. tit 63, §§ 3101-3111 (1985)	OKLAHOMA Statutes, Title 58, §§ 1051 1062		
OREGON Rev. Stat. §§ 97.050-.090 (1977)	OREGON Rev. Stat. §§ 126.407 & 126.413		OREGON Rev.Stat. § 97-083(2) amended H.B. 2963 (1983)
	PENNSYLVANIA * Statutes, Title 20 §§ 5601-5607		
	RHODE ISLAND Gen Laws § 34-22-6.1	RHODE ISLAND Gen Laws, §§ 23-4.10-1 - 4.10-2 (1986)	
SOUTH CAROLINA Code Ann. §§ 44-77-10 - 160 (1986)	SOUTH CAROLINA Code Ann. § 32-13-10		
	SOUTH DAKOTA Cod. Laws Ann. §§ 59-7- 2.1 - 59-7-4		
TENNESSEE Code Ann. §§ 32-11-101 - 110 (1985)	TENNESSEE Code Ann. §§ 34-13-101 - 34-13-108		

STATE LEGISLATION PROVIDING FOR:

NATURAL DEATH ACTS/ RIGHT TO DIE ACTS	DURABLE POWER OF ATTORNEY	DURABLE POWER OF ATTORNEY FOR HEALTH CARE	FAMILY CONSENT ACTS
TEXAS Health & Safety Code, art. 4590h (1977)	TEXAS Probate Code Ann. § 36A (1980)		TEXAS Civ. Stat. Art. 459 0h amended H.B. 403 (1985)
UTAH Code Ann. §§ 75-2-1101-1118 (1985)	UTAH Code Ann. §§ 75-5-501 & 502		UTAH Code Ann. § 78-14-5(4), §§ 75-2-1101-1118 (1985)
VERMONT Stat. Ann. Tit. 18, §§ 5251-5262 & Tit. 13, §§ 1801 (1982)	VERMONT Stat. Ann., Tit. 14 §§ 3051-3052		
VIRGINIA Code §§ 54-325. 8:1- 13 (1983)	VIRGINIA Code Ann. §§ 11-9.1 - 11-9.3		VIRGINIA Code Ann. § 54-325. 8.6 (1984)
WASHINGTON Rev. Code Ann. §§ 70.122.010 - .905 (1979)	WASHINGTON Rev. Code § 11.94.010		
WEST VIRGINIA Code §§ 16-30-1 - 10 (1984)	WEST VIRGINIA Code § 27-11-6		

STATE LEGISLATION PROVIDING FOR:

NATURAL DEATH ACTS/ RIGHT TO DIE ACTS	DURABLE POWER OF ATTORNEY	DURABLE POWER OF ATTORNEY FOR HEALTH CARE	FAMILY CONSENT ACTS
WISCONSIN Stat. Ann. §§ 154.01.-15 (1983)	WISCONSIN Statutes § 243.07		
WYOMING Statutes §§ 35-22-101 - 109 (1987)	WYOMING Statutes §§ 34-9-101 - 34-9-108		

* States where existing legislation for Durable Power of Attorney has been amended to provide for health care decisions.

** States where courts have addressed the issue of whether the Durable Power of Attorney can be used for health care decisions.

Source: Concern For Dying, 250 West 57th Street, New York, New York 10107, with additional information from public records.

Copies of state legislation, state directives to physicians, state durable power of attorney forms are available from Concern For Dying upon request.

Appendix 9

TWELVE QUESTIONS TO ANSWER BEFORE MAKING A
LIFE-SUSTAINING TREATMENT DECISION

1. Is the attending physician satisfied with the diagnostic and treatment procedures conducted to date?
2. Is the patient satisfied?
3. Is the patient mentally competent and emotionally ready to make a life-sustaining treatment decision?
4. Does the patient have enough information? Is the information in a form understandable to him or her?
5. When the patient is not able to make informed consent, is it clear *who* (physician or patient representative) has the right to make the decision? Is this a legal or a social/moral right? Are all parties aware of this distinction?
6. When another party is making the decision for the patient, are these factors taken into consideration: any earlier comment or requests made by the patient; the patient's religious preferences; the patient's philosophic beliefs? How has the patient responded to situations where others made similar decisions?
7. Do all members of the family agree with the decision?
8. Does the attending staff support the decision?
9. Have the legal requirements—hospital protocols, state laws, government regulations—been met?
10. Has the decision been documented in the chart?
11. Have the problems, and the resources brought to bear on these problems been recorded?
12. Has the decision maker received support from staff for the decision made?

When the answer is "no" to any of these questions, an intervention should be made. This might take any one of several forms:
• Other tests may need to be done.

- A psychologist, psychiatrist, social worker or other mental health personnel may need to be brought in to assess the patient and/or help explain the patient's preferences to others involved in the case.
- A chaplain, rabbi or clergyman may be needed to discuss or explain religious preferences.
- A clinically trained person may need to work with the feelings of family members or various staff people, regardless of whether the patient is the decision maker or not.
- Questions regarding the legal requirements and appropriate documentation may need to be answered.
- The decision maker should always receive support.

Appendix 10

DEFINITION OF HOSPITAL CODES

Code—Emergency effort to keep a patient breathing and his/her heart beating.

Calling a Code—Signaling for special personnel and equipment (a code or trauma team) to restore a patient's breathing and heartbeat, e.g., "Code Blue," "Doctor Blue."

No Code—Order for *no* emergency effort to restore breathing and heartbeat.

Modified Code—Order for certain life-sustaining treatments, but not others, e.g., drugs, but no intubation or CPR.

Extraordinary Means—"Heroic" efforts to keep a patient alive, e.g., calling a code; keeping a patient on a ventilator or kidney dialysis machine; use of a feeding tube.

Appendix 11

ORGAN DONATION CRITERIA

Many people would like to donate organs and tissues at the time of death, but don't know how to do it. Some states have passed Uniform Anatomical Gift Acts which allow individuals to fill out cards prior to death directly specifying the nature of their bequests. Families can also give permission, with or without the existence of a document signed by the deceased prior to death. However, organ donation can take place *only* when a patient has met the criteria of brain death. So the patient must be maintained on life-support machinery until transplant procedures can be put into place. Because nursing and medical staff are often too uncomfortable presenting these options to grieving relatives, and because relatives often don't know how to ask for such information, many donations that could occur simply do not happen. Also, due to the infrequency of these requests, staff may not have accurate information when asked.

The following are the tissue/organ donation criteria used by the Northern California Transplant Bank.

	Removal Time Limit (hours)	Age Limit of Donor (years)	Donation used for:
ORGAN:			
Heart	24	Newborn to 45	End-stage heart disease
Heart-Lung	24	12 to 45	End-stage cardiopulmonary disease
Heart Valves	24	Newborn to 55	Valve replacement
Kidney	24	1 month to 65	End-stage liver disease
TISSUE:			
Bone	24	15 to 55	Iliac crests & femurs; used in spinal fusions & non-union fractures

	Removal Time Limit (hours)	Age Limit of Donor (years)	Donation used for
TISSUE:			
Costal Cartilage	24	15 to 35	Facial reconstruction
Dura Mater	24	15 to 55	Surgical repairs of head injuries & reconstruction of middle ear
Eye	6-8	Newborn to 65 Over 65	Corneal transplants Medical research/training
Fascia Lata	24	15 to 55	Same use as dura mater
Middle Ear	24	15 to 55	Hearing repairs
Skin	24	15 to 55	Dressings for 3rd-degree burns
Tendons & Ligaments	24	15 to 45	Sports injury repairs

EXCLUSION FROM DONATION: Active infections and cancer. However, eye donations *are* accepted from patients with a history of cancer.

For more information, contact or have staff contact:
The Northern California Transplant Bank
2340 Clay Street, Suite 618   P.O. Box 7999
San Francisco, CA 94115   San Francisco, CA 94120
1 (800) 922-3100 (24-hour service)   (415) 922-3100

North American Transplant Coordinators Organization
1 (800) 24 DONOR or (412) 242-5378

A local Lion's Club or funeral home

Appendix 12

FUNERAL CHOICES

Most people tend to follow the customs of a community or the directions of a mortician without fully exploring funeral options. Here are the three basic choices and some facts about each that are not fully known or understood.

Earth Burial
- Immediate burials (within twenty-four hours) are much less expensive than burials that include embalming, viewing preparations, and funeral home use.
- In most states, embalming is *not* a legal requirement. Medical examiners and county coroners will know the law for your state.
- Refrigeration of the body until out-of-town relatives arrive to view the body is another less costly possibility. It is a little known option, and therefore rarely requested by families.

Cremation
- Most funeral homes can arrange for cremation, even if they don't provide the service on their premises.

Bequeathal to Science
- Arrangements must be made with the nearest medical school.
- Be sure to ascertain who will pay for the transportation costs—the medical school or the family.

Nonprofit memorial societies are the best sources of funeral information. They were organized by church and consumer groups to explore ways of offering simple, inexpensive, yet dignified funeral arrangements. They encourage their members to plan (but *not* pay) in advance. Through arrangements with various funeral directors throughout the country, they keep funeral costs lower for their members.

For information on the nearest nonprofit memorial society contact:

The Continental Association of Funeral and Memorial Societies
2001 "S" St. N.W.
Washington, D.C. 20009
(202) 462-8888

Also contact the Social Security Administration and the Veterans
Administration for burial benefits.

Appendix 13

SAMPLE
CARE PARTNER AGREEMENT

Patient: _____

Diagnosis: _____

Care Partner: _____

Relationship to Patient: _____

Professional Care Partner: _____

Care Partner's Available Days: _____

Care Partner's Available Hours: _____

Care Partner's Plan for Rest and Respite:

Patient's Plan for Care Partner(s):

Care Partner Tasks:	Person Responsible	Training Completed
1. _____	_____	_____
2. _____	_____	_____
3. _____	_____	_____
4. _____	_____	_____
5. _____	_____	_____

Appendix 14

EXAMPLES OF POSSIBLE CARE PARTNER TASKS

Nursing/Personal Care
Assist with menu selection
Assist with meals
Monitor IVs
Monitor or give medication
Give back rubs
Give manicures/pedicures
Apply compresses
Give baths
Change compresses
Change dressings
Flush catheters
Take temperature
Take blood pressure
Suction patient
Monitor ventilator/feeding bag
Clean gastric tube
Assist with ambulation
Give short wheelchair trips

Spiritual Care
Assist patient in participating
in any spiritual ritual or
worship of his/her choice
(e.g., prayer, meditation,
chanting, spiritual rites,
scripture readings)
Secure pastoral care/
spiritual counseling
as requested
Provide atmosphere that
respects dignity of the patient
Assist patient in finding
meaning in his/her
illness

Psycho-Social Care
Listen to patient
Read to patient
Bring music/movies to room
Bring decorations and
personal belongings to room
(e.g., family pictures, flowers,
balloons, stuffed animals,
artwork)
Move things around room
for visual interest
Bring favorite food or
condiments to patient

**Advocate/Patient
Representative**
Be in attendance during
rounds
Bring in specialists (e.g.,
Nutritionist, Health Educator)
Outline training needs of
patient or care partner
Inventory supplies and notify
appropriate staff of needs
Record patient progress/
comments in medical chart
Keep journal or hospital log
for patient or family

See that patient is comfortable (e.g., warmth, sound level, general courtesy)
Sit in silence in room
Check on house/apartment
Do household chores
Comfort other family members

Inform patient of his/her rights; help patient become his/her own advocate
Communicate for patient when *clearly* requested by patient; see that request is recorded in medical chart and understood by staff

Appendix 15

SAMPLE
HOSPITAL LOG

Date & Time	Procedure, Event or Information Given (Temperature, Blood Pressure, Lab Tests Done, Information Presented by Doctor or Nurse, Visitors, General Impression of the Day, Etc.)	Person Recording

BIBLIOGRAPHY

BOOKS

Bolen, Jean Shinoda. *The Tao of Psychology: Synchronicity and the Self.* New York: Harper and Row, 1978.

Brenner, Paul. *A Shared Creation: The Meaning of Pregnancy.* Dallas: Saybrook Publishing Co., 1988.

Cantor, Robert Chernin. *And a Time to Live: Toward Emotional Well-Being During the Crisis of Cancer.* New York: Harper and Row. 1978.

Castaneda, Carlos. *The Teaching of Don Juan: A Yaqui Way of Knowledge.* New York: Simon and Schuster, 1974.

Clifford, Denis. *The Power of Attorney Book.* Berkeley: Nolo Press, 1985.

Cousins, Norman. *Anatomy of an Illness as Perceived by the Patient: Reflections on Healing and Regeneration.* New York: W.W. Norton, 1979.

_____. *The Healing Heart: Antidotes to Panic and Helplessness.* New York: W.W. Norton, 1982.

Duda, Deborah. *A Guide to Dying at Home.* Sante Fe: John Muir Publications, 1982.

Foos-Graber, Anya. *Deathing: An Intelligent Alternative for the Final Moments of Life.* Reading, Mass.: Addison-Wesley Publishing Co., 1984.

Forrester, Victoria. "So Penetrant a Light" from *A Latch Against the Wind*. Copyright © 1985 Victoria Forrester. Reprinted with the permission of Atheneum Publishers, an imprint of MacMillan Publishing Company.

Frankl, Viktor E. *Man's Search for Meaning.* Boston: Beacon Press, 1939.

Fries, James and Lawrence M. Crapo. *Vitality and Aging.* San Francisco: W.H. Freeman and Co., 1981.

Garfield, Charles A. (ed.). *Stress and Survival: The Emotional Realities of Life-Threatening Illness.* St. Louis: C.V. Mosby Co., 1979.

Heron, Echo. *Intensive Care: The Story of a Nurse.* New York: Atheneum, 1987.

Hine, Virginia. *Last Letter to the Pebble People: "Aldie Soars."* Santa Cruz: Unity Press, 1977.

Inlander, Charles B. and Ed Weiner. *Take This Book to the Hospital With You.* Emmaus, Pa.: Rodale Press, 1985.

Jaffe, Dennis and Cynthia Scott. *From Burnout to Balance: A Workbook for Peak Performance and Self-Renewal.* New York: McGraw-Hill, 1984.

Jampolsky, Gerald. *Teach Only Love: The Seven Principles of Attitudinal Healing.* New York: Bantam Books, 1983.

Jonsen, Albert R., Mark Siegler and William Winslade. *Clinical Ethics: A Practical Approach to Ethical Decisions in Clinical Medicine.* New York: Macmillan Publishing Co., 1982.

Kalish, Richard. "The Effects of Death Upon the Family." *Death and Dying.* Leonard Pearson (ed.). Cleveland, Ohio: Case Western Reserve University, 1969.

Kastenbaum, Robert. "In Control." *Psychosocial Care of the Dying Patient.* Charles A. Garfield (ed.), New York: McGraw-Hill Book Company, 1978.

Koestenbaum, Peter. *The Heart of Business: Ethics, Power and Philosophy.* Dallas: Saybrook Publishing Co., 1987.

Kübler-Ross, Elisabeth. *To Live Until We Say Goodbye.* Englewood, N.J.: Prentice-Hall, 1978.

Lamott, Anne. *Hard Laughter.* New York: Viking Press, 1979.

LeBoyer, Frederick. "Interview with an Obstetrician." *Lilias, Yoga and Your Life.* Lilias Folan. New York: Macmillan Publishing Co., 1981.

LeBoyer, Frederick. *Birth Without Violence.* New York: Alfred A. Knopf, 1976.

Levine, Stephen. *Who Dies: An Investigation of Conscious Living and Conscious Dying.* New York: Anchor Press, 1982.

May, Rollo. *My Quest for Beauty.* Dallas: Saybrook Publishing Co., 1985.

_____, *The Meaning of Anxiety.* New York: Ronald Press Co., 1950.

McCoy, Marjorie Casebier. *To Die with Style!* Nashville: Abingdon Press, 1974.

Nouwen, Henri J. M. *The Wounded Healer: Ministry in Contemporary Society.* Garden City, New York: Image Books, 1972.

Ornish, Dean. *Stress, Diet and Your Heart.* New York: Holt, Rinehart and Winston, 1982.

Paul, Jordan and Margaret. *Do I Have to Give Up Me to Be Loved by You?* Minneapolis: CompCare Publications, 1983.

Peck, M. Scott. *People of the Lie: The Hope for Healing Human Evil.* New York: Simon and Schuster, 1983.

Peters, Tom. *In Search of Excellence.* New York: Harper and Row, 1982.

Peters, Tom. *A Passion for Excellence.* New York: Harper and Row, 1985.

Remen, Naomi. *The Human Patient.* Garden City, New York: Anchor Press/ Doubleday, 1980.

Rosenbaum, Peter and John Beebe. *Psychiatric Treatment: Crisis/Clinic/ Consultation.* New York: McGraw Hill, 1975.

Rossman, Martin L. *Healing Yourself: A Step-By-Step Program for Better Health Through Imagery.* New York: Walker and Co., 1987.

Siegel, Bernie S. *Love, Medicine and Miracles: Lessons Learned about Self-Healing from a Surgeon's Experience with Exceptional Patients.* New York: Harper and Row, 1986.

Simonton, O. Carl, Stephanie Matthews-Simonton and James Creighton. *Getting Well Again: A Step-By-Step, Self-Help Guide to Overcoming Cancer for Patients and their Families.* Los Angeles: J.P. Tarcher, Inc., 1978.

Stoddard, Sandol. *The Hospice Movement: A Better Way of Caring for the Dying.* Briarcliff Manor, N.Y.: Stein and Day, 1978.

Woodsen, Robert. "Hospice Care in Terminal Illness." *Psychosocial Care of the Dying Patient.* Charles A. Garfield (ed.). McGraw Hill Book Co: New York, 1978.

ARTICLES

Bateson, Mary Catherine. "Six Days of Dying." *The Co-Evolution Quarterly* (now *Whole Earth Review*) Winter (1980): 4-11.

Bergren, Wendy. "Mom Is Very Sick—Here's How to Help." *Focus on the Family* 6, no. 10 (November 1982): 4,5.

Brecher, John, with David T. Friendly, Frank Maier and Vincent Coppola. "Keeping the Patient in Stitches." *Newsweek* (August 1, 1982): 65.

Carey, John, with Jerry Buckley and Jennifer Smith. "Hospital Hospitality: Health Workers Learn to Treat Patients with Kindness." *Newsweek* (February 11, 1985): 78, 79.

Cohn, Victor. "So You Want Your Medical Records." *San Francisco Chronicle* (April 24, 1985): EE1.

Driver, Caroline. "What a Dying Man Taught Doctors About Caring." *Medical Economics* 50 (January 22, 1973): 81-86.

Fine, Louis L. "Emotional Management Seen As Crucial Element in Outcome of Pediatric Intensive Care." *Human Aspects of Anesthesia* (January/February 1985): 1,7.

Hamilton, Mildred. "An Innovative 'Care by Parent' Program." *San Francisco Examiner* (December 21, 1986): E4.

Hull, Jennifer Bingham. "Surviving a Stay in the Hospital, From Consent Forms to Discharge." *Wall Street Journal* (May 2, 1985): 31.

Klagsbrun, Samuel C. "Cancer, Emotions, and Nurses." *American Journal of Psychiatry* 126 (1970): 1237-1244.

Larsen, Dave. "The 'Ums' and 'Ahs' of Social Status: What Conversation Ploys Reveal." *San Francisco Chronicle* (December 24, 1984): 12.

"Ruth Hoffman." *San Francisco Chronicle* (August 11, 1973): 4.

Stier, Richard. "The Economics of Patient Satisfaction: How to Deliver Shockingly Good Customer Service at a Substantial Profit." *Healthcare Forum* (September/October 1987): 19, 20.

Tallmer, Louise and Barbara Ribakove. "Co-op Care Arrives." *Family Health* (now *Health, The Magazine for Total Well-Being*) 1, no. 6 (March 1980): 20.

Wacker, Ronnie. "The Good Die Younger." *San Francisco Chronicle* (November 25, 1985): 20, 22.

PAMPHLETS/BOOKLETS/DOCUMENTS

A Spirit Soars: Beyhan's Journey. Tom Pinkson (Project Coordinator), Box 591, Forest Knolls, CA. 94933. (Booklet)

Guidelines for Implementation of AB—610: Patient Access to Medical Records. California Medical Record Association, Inc., (October 1982). (Booklet)

Planetree Model Hospital Project. Robin Orr (Project Administrator), 2040 Webster Street, San Francisco, CA. 94115. (Pamphlet)

President's Commission for the Study of Ethical Problems in Medicine and Biomedical and Behavioral Research. Deciding to Forego Life-Sustaining Treatment: A Report on the Ethical, Medical, and Legal Issues in Treatment Decisions (March 1983) U.S. Government Printing Office, Washington, D.C. 20402. (Document)

Sarath, Maria, Melissa Auerbach and Ted Bogue. *Medical Records: Getting Yours: A Consumer's Guide to Obtaining Your Medical Records* (1980). Health Research Group, 2000 "P" Street, N.W., Suite 708, Washington, D.C. 20036. (Booklet)

Ronnie Wacker. "The Good Die Younger." © 1985 *San Francisco Chronicle*. Used with permission of the *San Francisco Chronicle*.

CHAPTER FIVE

Norman Cousins. *Anatomy of an Illness: As Perceived by the Patient.* © 1979 Norman Cousins. Used with permission of W. W. Norton & Company, Inc.

Rollo May. *My Quest for Beauty.* © 1985 Rollo May. Used with permission of the Saybrook Publishing Company.

Dean Ornish. *Stress, Diet and Your Heart.* © 1982 Dean Ornish. Used with permission of Henry Holt and Company, Inc.

"Ruth Hoffman." © 1973 *San Francisco Chronicle*. Used with permission of the *San Francisco Chronicle*.

CHAPTER SIX

A Spirit Soars: Beyhan's Journey. Tom Pinkson (Project Coordinator), Box 591, Forest Knolls, CA 94933. Used with permission of Tom Pinkson.

Wendy Bergren. "Mom is Very Sick: Here's How to Help," *Focus on the Family*, © November, 1982. All rights reserved. Used with permission of Scott Bergren and *Focus on the Family*.

Jordan and Margaret Paul. *Do I Have to Give Up Me to Be Loved by You?* © 1983 Jordan and Margaret Paul. Used with permission of CompCare Publishers.

Peter Rosenbaum and John Beebe. *Psychiatric Treatment: Crisis/Clinic/Consultation.* © Peter Rosenbaum and John Beebe. Used with permission of C. Peter Rosenbaum and McGraw-Hill Company.

CHAPTER SEVEN

Jean Shinoda Bolen. *The Tao of Psychology: Synchronicity and the Self.* © 1978 Jean Shinoda Bolen. Used with permission of Harper & Row Publishers, Inc.

Louis L. Fine. "Emotional Management Seen As Crucial Element in Outcome of Pediatric Intensive Care." © 1985 *Human Aspects of Anesthesia*. Used with permission of McMahon Publishing.

APPENDIX

"Example of a Living Will," Reprinted with permission of Concern for Dying, 250 West 57th Street, New York 10107; (212) 246–6962.

"Patient's Bill of Rights," © 1972 American Hospital Association. Reprinted with permission of the American Hospital Association.

"Patient Rights in a Nursing Home," Reprinted from *A Consumer Guide to Nursing Homes*, Department of Health Services, Licensing and Certification Division, 714 "P" Street, Sacramento, CA 95814. [Taken from California Code of Regulations, Title 22, Social Security, Division 5, Licensing and Certification of Health Facilities and Referral Agencies, Chapter 3, Section 72527(a).]

INDEX

acupressure/acupuncture 185
against medical advice (AMA)
    79
agreement, care partner
    helping the "helper" 147, 148
    sample form 23, 282
    verbal 26
    while under anesthesia 117,
        118
    written 22, 23, 69, 70, 117, 118
aikido 102
Aird, John C. 237
Albert Einstein Medical Center,
    Philadelphia 232, 233
American Cancer Society 169
American Civil Liberties Union
    81
American Journal of Psychiatry
    220–223
American Medical Association
    81
American Medical Records
    Association 81
American Network 232
American Red Cross 169
Anatomy of an Illness 113
And a Time to Live 201
"Anderson Network," M.D.
    Anderson Hospital and
    Tumor Institute, University of
    Texas, Houston 165
anesthesia
    patient's instructions before
        118
    reducing the effects of 179
Annas, George 81
Asklepia 239–240
assertive communication skills
    84–102
    avoiding overkill 100–102

"broken-record" 86–87
"fogging" 86
assertion and longevity studies
    72
Association of Humanistic
    Psychology 220

Baker, Edward Thomas 187–188
Barber, Dr. Neil 188, 198
Bartlett, Edward 81
Bateson, Gregory 73, 185
Bateson, Mary Catherine 73
Beebe, Dr. John 173
Bergren, Wendy 156
bioethical
    committees 191–193
    conference 197
Birth Without Violence 72
Bolen, Dr. Jean Shinoda 185,
    241, 242
Boston Globe, The 242
Brenner, Dr. Paul 69, 143, 144,
    172
Browning, Rosa, "Get Well
    Project" 107, 108
"burn-out," *see Concept Index,*
    IV
    among family members
        153–163
    among professionals 75,
        139–144
    care partner approach to
        139–144
    institution's responsibility for
        prevention 145–147

Cantor, Dr. Robert Chernin
    201

297

informed consent 78
imaging 50, 51, 111, 112, 121
insurance statistics and
   companies 38, 47
St. Paul Fire and Marine
   Insurance Company 38
intensive care unit 176–186
   pediatric 181, 182
intuition and healing 186
Ireland Corporation 229

Jaffe, Dennis 156
Jewish-sponsored support
   programs 169
Jonsen, Albert R. 242

Kaiser, Lee 229
Kalish, Dr. Richard 227
Karuk medicine man, Red Hawk
   148
Kastenbaum, Dr. Robert 41
Kelly, Dr. James 180
Klagsbrun, Dr. Samuel 220–223
Koestenbaum, Dr. Peter 39
Kübler-Ross, Dr. Elisabeth 73,
   225

Lamott, Anne 172
Last Letter to the Pebble People 172
Latch Against the Wind, A 103
LeBoyer, Dr. Frederick 72, 185
L'Engle, Madeleine 172
legislation
   giving patients the right to
      access medical records
      255–259
   providing for living will,
      natural death acts, durable
      power of attorney, family
      consent acts 268–275

Levin, Lowell 71, 88
Levine, Stephen 179
life support decisions, *see*
   Concept Index, VII
   care partner approach
      190–191, 194–213
   problems of present system
      73, 187–190, 191–194
   twelve questions to answer
      before making 276, 277
listening skills 92–95
living will
   example of 263
   definition, advantages,
      drawbacks of 264
log book, *see hospital log book*
Love, Medicine and Miracles 112
Lowman, Beyhan 134–135, 138

MacLaine, Shirley 115
malpractice suits,
   cause of 193, 197
   ways to reduce claims 37,
      192
Man's Search for Meaning 50
Marriott Corporation 231, 232
Matthews-Simonton, Stephanie
   111
May, Rollo 110, 162, 163
Meaning of Anxiety, The 162
medical charts, *see charts*
medical records, *see charts*
Medical Economics 108
medicare 37
meditation 122
"Mom Is Very Sick—Here's
   How to Help" 155, 156
Montana, Joe 115
Mother Teresa 161, 234
music
   importance for healing and
      stimulation 116